Leading
Change

Transformational

The Physician-Executive Partnership

Leading
Transformational
Change

The Physician-Executive Partnership

Thomas A. Atchison
Joseph S. Bujak

Health Administration Press
Chicago, Illinois

This publication is intended to provide accurate and authoritative information in regard to the subject matter covered. It is sold, or otherwise provided, with the understanding that the publisher is not engaged in rendering professional services. If professional advice or other expert assistance is required, the services of a competent professional should be sought.

The statements and opinions contained in this book are strictly those of the author(s) and do not represent the official positions of the American College of the Healthcare Executives or of the Foundation of the American College of Healthcare Executives.

05   04   03   02   5   4   3   2

Library of Congress Cataloging-in-Publication Data

Atchison, Thomas A., 1945–
    Leading transformational change : the physician-executive partnership/
    Thomas A. Atchison, Joseph S. Bujak.
        p. ; cm.
    Includes bibliographical references.
    ISBN 1-56793-161-8
    1. Physician executives. 2. Health services administration.
    I. Bujak, Joseph S. II. Title.
    [DNLM: 1. Organizational Innovation—United States. 2. Administrative
Personnel—United States. 3. Health Care Reform—United States. 4. Health Care
Sector—trends—United States. 5. Interprofessional Relations—United States. 6.
Physician's Role—United States. WA 540 AA1863L 2001]
    RA971 .A879 2001
    362.1'068—dc21   2001026487
                                                                                        CIP

The paper used in this publication meets the minimum requirements of American National Standard for Information Sciences–Permanence of Paper for Printed Library Materials, ANSI Z39.48-1984. ∞ ™

Editor: Diana Flynn; Cover design: Betsy Perez.

Health Administration Press
A division of the Foundation of the
    American College of Healthcare Executives
1 North Franklin Street, Suite 1700
Chicago, IL 60606-3491
(312) 424-2800

CONTENTS

PREFACE

HEALTHCARE IS AN industry characterized by constant and unpredictable change. Payment issues, access problems, technology improvements, breakthrough pharmaceuticals, and shifting population needs are some of the most common factors affecting delivery. The consequences of this reality are most readily experienced by practicing physicians. All of these dramatic shifts in the healthcare industry require fundamental changes in the way hospitals and health systems relate to physicians.

The economics of healthcare delivery dominates boardrooms and executive suites across the nation. The key variable in the revenue and expense patterns of any healthcare enterprise is the way physicians practice medicine. Several models have been developed in an attempt to "control" physician practice patterns. Schemes such as buying practices, using benchmarked productivity measures, and assigning risk to physicians have resulted in varying degrees of failure. This text grew out of our attempt to identify the core reasons for these failures.

The historical relationship between physicians and the hospitals in which they practice no longer remains beneficial to either party. Health corporations, payers, and consumers challenge physician independence. Physicians view the changing healthcare environment as a threat to their power (e.g., to make clinical decisions) and control (e.g., their ability to run their practices). Health delivery systems have viewed the last several years as an opportunity ("at last") to create business models that shift the power and control of patient care, and the subsequent revenues, to them. Business models focus only on the tangible aspects of physician behavior. The common metrics of tangible business practices are tied to money, sources of funds, and use of funds.

The thesis of this book is that while profitability is important, business models are inappropriate and have proven to be ineffective in working with physicians. The alternative presented falls under the category of building physician partnerships. The most important contributors to successful partnerships between healthcare systems and physicians are the intangibles of physician behavior. Business models typically focus on surface issues using linear economic models. The partnership model described in this book focuses on the deeper dimensions of physician performance using nonlinear change management methodologies. The goal of this approach is not to diminish the importance of tangibles, but rather to demonstrate that the intangibles are equally important. This text will describe the main intangibles contributing to successful partnerships, expose some common and flawed assumptions about physicians, differentiate the characteristics of an expert culture (physicians) and a collective culture (nonphysicians), and provide a developmental model for change management with physicians.

Chapter 1 sets the tone for the need for a new model of partnership with physicians. Chapter 2 discusses several operating assumptions, the flaws of which create a toxic work environment. Chapter 3 introduces the essential dynamic of change management, which is that our perceptions control our behavior. Chapter 4 introduces the difference between experts and collectives and explains why an understanding of the difference between these two populations is required to select those interventions that align physicians and those that align collectives. Chapter 5 maintains that changes in the healthcare industry to date are small compared to those that will occur in the future. Tenets found in complexity science are used to help understand future possibilities. Chapter 6 reinforces the message in most organizational change texts—leadership is the key. Chapter 7 discusses the need for trust to become a strategic prerequisite to partnering with physicians. Chapter 8 reviews the critical need to measure those elements that are being managed. Chapter 9 describes the developmental model and defines the 24 elements that affect change management. Chapter 10 is a summary of the need to focus on the intangibles to create and strengthen partnerships with physicians.

We hope that you find this text enjoyable to read and useful in all aspects of improvement in physician relations.

Thomas A. Atchison, Ed.D.
Joseph S. Bujak, M.D., FACPE

Chapter One

HEALTHCARE: A TRANSFORMING INDUSTRY

"...the task is not so much to see what no one yet has seen, but to think what nobody has yet thought about that which everybody sees."

Arthur Schopenhauer

T HE HEALTHCARE INDUSTRY is experiencing profound transformational changes. During times of such change, fundamental beliefs, roles, relationships, and behaviors are challenged. A sense of security and predictability disappears. Challenges to historical paradigms are causing healthcare providers to become anxious and unhappy. Control of the healthcare industry has shifted to payers, regulators, and consumers. Consequently, the culture of the provider community is in chaos, and professional dissatisfaction is increasing. The professional half-life of healthcare executives is becoming progressively shorter. Physicians no longer encourage their children to become physicians, and nurses are in short supply. The sense of joy and happiness is disappearing from the healthcare workplace.

1

In response to these challenges, healthcare organizations sought to aggregate for leverage. They viewed patients as a commodity and resented profit margins accruing to third-party administrators. Coming together, they believed, would increase negotiating power and prevent the further loss of control.

Attention focused on altering structure and "doing the deal." Mergers and acquisitions became commonplace for healthcare organizations. Physicians began to aggregate by forming larger groups or selling their practices to healthcare organizations or for-profit physician management companies. Simply creating the proper organizational structure was believed to result in necessary behavioral changes. Little time was spent defining the what and the why of the new enterprises, and often, when physicians were involved, political realities prompted healthcare organizations to be all-inclusive. Integrated delivery systems were formed to deny profit to the insurance industry and to control the elusive continuum of care. Providers sought to acquire economic risk despite having no experience with managing risk or any infrastructure that would successfully support such an effort. The hospital's focus was on controlling the system and in creating geographical distribution channels. Attempts to involve physicians led to the formation of physician hospital organization (PHOs), management services organizations (MSOs), or physician employment. However, most of the time integrated delivery systems remained merely holding companies. New corporate structures rarely created the anticipated benefits, almost never successfully integrated the strengths of the contributing cultures and, therefore, failed to realize the hoped for synergies. Physicians believed that their position was protected by medical licensure. They sought to preserve their income and autonomy and focused on generating revenue from the application of ancillary services.

Almost every attempt of hospital organizations to partner with physicians has failed. The strategies of purchasing practices and employing physicians have not improved patient care and have been business failures. Physician management companies are disappearing. No measurement of integrated success was found in forming integrated delivery systems. As a result, the various stakeholders have consciously or unconsciously entered into zero sum games of economic self–interest.

In this chapter we will discuss how to adapt to transformational change. Factors driving change include the accelerating pace of new technology in healthcare, the changing structure of modern organizations, and the compression of time and space. A look at the traditions of healthcare and why people have historically entered the profession will also shed some light on the future of healthcare in this world of profound change.

INTERDEPENDENCY

Are successful healthcare organizations dependent on their associated medical staff? The answer is an emphatic yes. "Healthcare CEOs can't cross the great divide where structure is determined by professional standards and technological imperatives, not administrative dictates" (Mintzberg and Glouberman 1999) Physicians allocate almost all of the direct costs that attend patient care, and with traditional sources of reimbursement becoming fixed, controlling costs becomes the primary way to create a positive operating margin. In the absence of a cooperative relationship with physicians, the healthcare organization cannot survive economically.

Conversely, are physicians dependent on healthcare organizations for their success? This question is more difficult to answer. Intensivists, acute care specialists, and those physicians requiring access to very expensive technology remain tied to the acute care hospital setting. However, the advent of hospitalists and full-time emergency room physicians has made it possible and economically advantageous for primary care physicians to rarely come to the hospital. Many specialty physicians have taken advantage

3

of advancing technology and perform technical procedures in their own offices or in free-standing ambulatory surgery centers.

The forces that are transforming the healthcare marketplace are demanding that physicians aggregate. The regulatory environment, the growing complexity and cost of managing the business side of clinical practice, and the expanding knowledge and complexity of clinical medicine require access to information and support systems that most independent physicians cannot afford. Physicians desire to fashion some economies of scale, to simplify processes, and to create some time, the most precious of all deliverables. Most physicians need to partner with an organization that can be a source of necessary capital, if for no other reason than to have access to the necessary information that will enable them to practice efficient and effective patient care and to remain in regulatory compliance.

Other than some single-specialty or procedure-focused successes, most physician attempts to align with venture capitalists, stock-owned companies, and other for-profit organizations have failed. Achieving an adequate return on investment creates an environment that challenges physician autonomy and generates professional dissatisfaction. Although not-for-profits theoretically share the same principles and purposes that align with the most deeply held values of the medical profession, most broad-based attempts to create healthcare organization-physician ventures have failed as well. Healthcare organizations and physicians are interdependent for their success. Failure to cooperate does not remove the interdependency; rather, it makes it toxic.

HOW TO ADAPT TO TRANSFORMATIONAL CHANGE

Gaining insight is the first step toward successful adaptation. To be the author of your future, you need to travel the following journey:

- understand the dynamic forces that are driving transformational change;
- reaffirm the essence of who you are and revisit your founding story to reconfirm both your personal and/or organizational sense of purpose; and
- take responsibility for creating your own future (Arbuckle 1995).

It is essential to understand your operating assumptions and to reaffirm that they remain valid in light of a significantly changing environment. If they are no longer valid, changing those assumptions and letting go of failing paradigms is a critical step toward engaging change and creating your own future.

DYNAMIC FORCES

A number of forces are transforming the healthcare industry. These include:

- global economic competition;
- a shifting emphasis away from an acute care model of delivery towards a chronic disease management model;
- a growing emphasis on wellness and prevention;
- focus on the consumer;
- advancing technology;
- increasing competition; and
- the emergence of the "new economy."

The global economy. In no other country do businesses allocate so significant a portion of their overhead providing healthcare benefits for their employees. Because of global competition, the unpredictable and uncontrollable increments in the cost of U. S. healthcare benefits have become intolerable. This reality coincided with Dr. Jack Wennberg's publications describing the variation with which medical services are provided across different geographical regions (Wennberg 1987).

In reviewing healthcare data and using a process termed "small area analysis of variation," Doctor Wennberg was able to document the wide variation with which healthcare services are applied. For example, a patient's likelihood of undergoing a transurethral resection of the prostate gland, having a hysterectomy, or dying either in a hospital or at home varied dramatically from one area to another, such as the university hospital settings of Boston and New Haven and smaller, geographically proximate towns in New England. Analogous studies have been replicated on a national level and have culminated in the publication of the *Dartmouth Atlas* (Wennberg 1996). This publication geographically correlates the frequency with which health care services are applied with the medical resources available and the demographics of the area. Widespread geographical variations exist across the United States. Are patients in one area being over treated, or are some patients being undertreated? How do we assess the value of what payers are buying? When the healthcare provider community failed to respond to these questions, employers turned to health maintenance organization (HMOs) and managed care organizations to help them control healthcare costs.

Chronic disease management. The United States' healthcare industry is built on an acute model of care delivery. When individuals are acutely ill, they need access to physicians and hospitals. Providers are like mechanics who fix things that are broken. Currently, however, the majority of healthcare encounters are for chronic and not acute problems. When you are chronically ill, you primarily need access to information.

Numerous studies have documented how an interested patient, when provided with relevant information, can produce medical outcomes that are superior to those of traditional physician management practices. This is true for diseases like childhood

6

asthma, hypertension, diabetes, congestive heart failure, and os-teoarthritis. As a result, physicians are less essential to the management process and are being usurped by physician extenders, insurers, or the patients themselves. Case management, disease management, and other attempts to integrate the continuum of medical care are additional examples of this changing emphasis. Self-diagnosis and self-therapy are significant trends today.

The wellness model. The healthcare industry is also shifting from a sickness model to a wellness model reflected in an expanding interest in alternative and complementary medicine. Print and broadcast media extensively cover subjects that relate to health maintenance, quality of life, and longevity. The industry that surrounds exercise, vitamins, food supplements, and dieting similarly demonstrate a growing emphasis on longevity and quality of life. An enhanced concern for the quality of the environment reflects an appreciation for how environmental factors contribute to ill health. Health in the workplace initiatives and integrated approaches towards workman's compensations provide additional examples. Although wellness for the most part is not supported by health insurance, it is supported by discretionary spending and is part of the growing consumer movement in the United States.

The consumer movement.[1] A growing consumer movement has emerged in the healthcare industry, and the healthcare provider no longer has control of it (Herzlinger 1997). Although allopathic healthcare is still largely organized for the convenience of the provider, the healthcare industry has recently begun to focus on the needs of the patient/consumer. Historically, patients relinquished their healthcare needs to their physician. Now, the baby boomer generation wants to be in control of managing its own healthcare needs. They seek advice, counsel, and partnership with their healthcare providers and would prefer to make health decisions jointly.

7

Just as the attitude of consumers is changing, copayments and deductibles are increasing and healthcare has begun to act more like a traditional market. More of the increased cost of healthcare is being borne by the consumer. There is less of a disconnect between the payer of services and the consumer of those services. In order to compete, providers are discovering the need to create a distinctive identity that differentiates them in the marketplace and to provide value to the customer.

Healthcare providers must begin to create value as perceived by the customer, and leave behind a one-size-fits-all approach. For example, different constituents have different needs and expectations and require access to different kinds of providers. The illnesses, needs, and expectations of the Medicare population are significantly different from those of an indemnity population, which in turn are different from those of a Medicaid population. In other service industries different delivery models provide services that meet different customer needs. In the hotel industry, for example, Marriott owns the Ritz-Carlton hotels, the Fairfield Inn hotels, and other varieties in between. Each division has different management and goals. An approach that successfully meets the needs of those who stay at the Fairfield Inn would never be successful in meeting the expectations of those who stay at the Ritz-Carlton. By contrast, in healthcare a single delivery system is presumed to meet the needs of different populations.

Advancing technology. Advancing technology is progressively moving the delivery site of healthcare services closer to the patient's home. Who would have imagined that ten years ago patients could undergo joint surgery or cholecystectomy with less than a one day stay in the hospital? The advent of laparoscopic surgery has markedly influenced the recovery time for many operative procedures. Similarly, polio vaccines have relegated iron lungs to museums, and psychotropic medications have transformed the approach to treating mental illness (Herzlinger 1997).

Increasing competition. Increasing competition is transforming the healthcare landscape. Not only is there an excess (and/or maldistribution) of physicians and hospital beds, but also a growing presence of allied health professionals and providers of alternative and complementary healthcare services. The secure economic position and the vested authority that once characterized physicians and hospitals are being challenged. Many businesses that have not traditionally been involved in the healthcare industry have begun to compete for portions of the healthcare dollar. The outsourcing of support functions reflects this dynamic. Advancing knowledge and the technology that underlies developing pharmaceutical, immunologic, and genetic interventions are transforming roles and traditional hierarchies.

The new economy.[2] The accelerating pace of change, instantaneous access to information and new knowledge, changing organizational structures, prosumption, disintermediation, deconstruction, and the compression of time and space are phenomena that are inherent to the information age and are affecting all industries including healthcare.

ACCELERATING PACE OF CHANGE

The information revolution is affecting the healthcare industry just as it has affected most other industries. A networked economy, referred to as the new economy, is significantly different from the industrial economy (Kelly 1998). Whereas the industrial economy is rooted in the production of things, the new economy focuses on intangibles like ideas, information, and relationships. The accelerating pace of change and the almost immediate access to information creates positive feedback loops in which every new idea and innovation becomes a springboard on which to build. The pace of change is asymptotic, that is, it progresses at an exponential rate, and the doubling time of change requires

9

only the square root of the antecedent interval (Russell 1998). We are at point where significance precedes momentum and where creativity is far more important than perfectibility. In this rapidly changing world it is more important to do the right thing than to continue to do the same thing better.

Since the future is unknowable, organizations require a pluralistic approach for strategic planning. It is not possible to create or buy all the knowledge and skill required to prepare for so many potential realities. This underlies the trend toward creating virtual organizations, alliances, and outsourcing, as leaderships seek to position their organizations for sustainability in an unknowable future. Robust adaptive strategies sacrifice apparent certainty for flexibility and a higher probability of success (Beinhocker 1999). Networking expands sourcing and distribution options while fixed investment and skill requirements fall.

ACCESS TO INFORMATION

Relationships in the industrial economy have been challenged by the separation of the economics of physical things from the economics of information (Evans and Wurster 2000). Every business is a compromise between the two. When a physical thing is sold, the owner ceases to own it. When information is sold, the seller still possesses it and is able to sell it again. Physical things are replicated at the cost of manufacturing. Information can be replicated at almost no additional cost and without limit. The economics of things are subject to laws of either diminishing or increasing returns. For example, diminishing returns occur when doubling the number of workers on a farm does not double the output of the land. Increasing returns are reflected in circumstances where economies of scale can be applied to the production of incremental quantities of product. Information obeys the law of perfectly increasing returns; that is, every time you double the number of applications of learned information, you reduce by one-half the cost of obtaining that information.

A huge disparity exists in healthcare in the amount of information available to the producer and consumer. Patients must navigate a convoluted maze in an attempt to reconstruct their medical history and to synthesize their medical information. Consequently, patients are at a disadvantage in their relationship with their provider who thereby occupies a position of power. Once consumers can access all of their relevant information, they will no longer be prisoners of the physical healthcare non-system. Patients will have the capacity to seek consultation and advice independent of geographical restrictions. The creation of a standardized electronic medical record will challenge the very notion of geographically based licensure and will challenge the current structure and function of healthcare delivery (Evans and Wurster 2000).

Summarizing available information. The current healthcare environment is characterized by a wealth of information. However, where an abundance of information exists there is a corresponding poverty of attention (Kelly 1998). How do you judge the quality of the information or even discover how to access the information? The proliferation of indexed newsletters represents one response to this challenge. For example, physicians cannot possibly read all of the published medical literature that relates to their area of medical practice. Therefore, they frequently subscribe to monthly publications that summarize a number of specialty journals. These abstracting services focus the physician's attention. Many similar ventures that help navigate the maze of available information are emerging and serve as a kind of *Consumer's Report*, summarizing and evaluating the overwhelming amount of available information.

In an analogous way, healthcare consumers have at their disposal an infinite variety of information through the print and broadcast media, as well as the Internet. It is difficult to interpret the validity and application of so much information, and consumers become dependent on intermediary businesses to direct them to the appropriate sources of information and frequently to draw conclusions on their behalf.

CHANGING ORGANIZATIONAL STRUCTURES

Healthcare is still primarily being provided in a preindustrial model. Physicians practice as artisans or guild members. Movements to bring healthcare to an industrial model include mergers and acquisitions, the hiring of physicians, the creation of integrated delivery systems, and the application of principles of industrial process control. In many ways this is an attempt to create economies of scale within an environment of shrinking reimbursement. While healthcare becomes industrialized, already industrialized industries are moving beyond an industrial model toward mass customization and a focused intent to satisfy individual consumer needs in response to expectations generated by expanded access to information.

In healthcare financing, this information age dynamic is reflected in the increasing rejection of the HMO model and the emergence of point-of-service insurance plans as the preferred customer alternative. The American public has rejected the strategy of payers to channel patients to contracted providers. This too reflects how customers and not providers are now in control of shaping the evolving healthcare industry. Healthcare consumers want to partner with their caregivers on their own terms. In an industrial economy, producers are in control; in an information economy, consumers are in control. In effect, the healthcare industry is moving through its version of the industrial revolution and the information revolution simultaneously.

In the new economy, relationships and context are replacing structure as the vehicle for supporting organizational success. In the industrial economy, hierarchy was necessary for mass production. Span of control was critical to moving information from the top down and for ensuring accountability from the bottom up. Today relevant real-time information can be made available to everyone. This allows for the flattening of organizations, the empowerment of line workers, and the ability to rapidly meet demands for enhanced efficiency and effectiveness of performance in response to the changing needs of customers.

PRODUCTION AND CONSUMPTION

Within the new economy the phenomenon of "prosumption" is occurring. Prosumption is a combination of two words—production and consumption. It refers to the blurring of the distinction between the producer of products and services and the primary consumer. For example, when using an ATM machine does a person work for the bank or are they a customer? When filling their gas tank, are people customers or do they work for the filling station? If they do a home pregnancy test, are they a patient or do they work for the obstetrician? Self-service often creates not only a more efficient operation, but also one that is attended by higher degrees of customer satisfaction. Online banking and catalog shopping are activities in which the customer is free to engage the business at his or her convenience. Those organizations that forge close ties with their customers are more likely to be successful in a consumer-driven economy.

Historically, physicians had a marked advantage over their patients with respect to medical information and knowledge. Now, however, patients frequently confront the doctor with printouts from the Internet and challenge him or her to respond to new considerations. The evening news heralds the results of the "latest and greatest" medical discovery before the physician has even unwrapped the journal in which it was published. Prosumption will become a part of maintaining customer loyalty in healthcare.

DISINTERMEDIATION

Disintermediation is another consequence of the information revolution. Disintermediation refers to bypassing the middleman.

ATM machines have disintermediated bank cashiers. Retail catalogs and factory outlet stores have disintermediated retail shops. Historically, middlemen served to bridge the information gap between the producer of goods or services and the customer. For example, electronics stores help shoppers evaluate the array of available electronic products. Now, customers can go directly to a computer manufacturer via the Internet and are no longer dependent on retail stores to help them purchase a personal computer. In a similar way, Schwab.com is disintermediating Merrill-Lynch by allowing individuals to personally trade stocks without the intercession of a traditional stockbroker. In an analogous fashion, 1-800-Dial-A-Nurse triage services and case management initiatives are disintermediating physicians from the doctor-patient relationship.

DECONSTRUCTION[3]

Deconstruction refers to disassembling, bypassing, or eliminating historically linked components of the business enterprise. A healthcare organization can deconstruct along the vertical links of its supply chain as when pharmaceutical firms directly market their products to the public. Similarly, information can be segregated into businesses in their own right such as WebMD.com. Intraorganizational relationships can be deconstructed by outsourcing medical transcription, housekeeping, or cafeteria services or decentralizing the registration process.

The community hospital is also vulnerable to deconstruction by providers of niche services. A hospital is an aggregation of a number of different service lines. Some of the service lines are significantly profitable, while others are marginally profitable or lose revenue. Because all of these service lines are aggregated into a single bottom line, each must compete for progressively diminishing capital resources. Producers of niche services have a sharper focus and are not distracted by having to compete with others service lines for resources. The growth of physician-owned ambulatory surgery centers that capture a significant portion of one of the healthcare organization's highest margin service lines is an example of how the aggregated system is being deconstructed by a horizontally integrated service line. Urgent care centers and the migration of ophthalmologic, endoscopic, and arthroscopic procedures into physician-owned facilities provide additional examples.

Healthcare organizations must deconstruct themselves. Although hospitals and healthcare systems consider other full-service healthcare organizations as their primary competitors, they are most vulnerable to those focused providers who can steal a significant percentage of their highest margin service lines. Once a value chain begins to deconstruct in this way, it is perilous to cling to the old business model. It is imperative that organizations begin to deconstruct themselves (Evans and Wurster 2000). One common example of this occurs when local surgeons begin to consider building their own outpatient surgery center. In response to this threat, many hospitals or health systems have chosen to willingly deconstruct themselves by developing joint ventures with those very same surgeons in an attempt to both preserve their relationship with the surgeons and to capture at least some of the profit margin that attends that service line. Fifty percent of something is preferable to one hundred percent of nothing. However, deconstructing an established business is not easy (Evans and Wurster 2000). Underestimating the requirements for acquiring new capabilities and overestimating the value of existing capabilities is a common trap.

COMPRESSION OF TIME AND SPACE[4]

Advancing technology and the information revolution are causing a compression of time and space (Zimmerman and Plsek 1998). In healthcare we moved from discovery to entitlement overnight. The public is instantly made aware of outcomes of the latest medical studies and an almost instant demand for its application is created. The amount of time it takes to make available new pharmaceutical drugs has been shortened. The advent of laparoscopic surgery has shortened both postoperative hospital stays and time for functional recovery. Space is also being compressed. For example, once all medical imaging is digitized, what will happen to the persons and space currently required to develop, catalog, store, and retrieve x-ray film? The accelerating pace of change implies that optimization will not last long. By the time you discover how to do something right, it no longer matters. A new technology has displaced the old.

REVISITING YOUR FOUNDING STORY

What are the roots and traditions of healthcare professions? How can those founding and essential principles endure in a world of profound change? Where does one find stability when the future is unknowable? Is the growing discontent within healthcare a manifestation of a failure to preserve the essence of what has historically been a calling rather than a job, a profession rather than a trade?

In a rapidly changing environment, sustainability is rooted in shared purpose and values and in rediscovering meaning and purpose in work (Collins and Porras 1997; Frankl 1984). The majority of physicians chose medicine as a career because of a desire to help others. However, during medical training an emphasis on science, deductive reasoning, and technology shifted the emphasis away from healing and toward curing. The doctor-patient relationship shifted to a doctor-disease or a doctor-technology relationship. The means became an end in itself.

Providers are being paid less for each unit of service provided. To maintain a targeted income, physicians have chosen to see more patients or produce more units of productivity. This shrinking unit-based reimbursement, combined with increasing specialization in medicine, have caused many healthcare providers to see patients in transactional ways. They view patients as units of production.

Although patients often desire to be listened to and touched, physicians frequently substitute impersonalized technology. The average time it takes for a physician to interrupt a patient's answer after soliciting their chief complaint is less than 20 seconds. Focusing on the disease and not the patient leaves the patient unsatisfied. A failure to "connect" with patients partially explains the growing popularity of alternative and complementary medicine. Many nontraditional providers emphasize a holistic and individualized approach.

Rediscovering the joy in work.[5] If caregivers are to experience meaning and purpose in their work they have to interact with patients in transformational and not transactional ways. Attentive listening and a desire to discover the context of illness creates a relationship that is far more intimate, personalized, enriching, and fulfilling. Arnold Relman, editor emeritus of the *New England Journal of Medicine,* stated that when physician satisfaction was at its all time high physicians were earning about three times the average income of other workers in the United States. Today, physicians earn approximately ten times this amount and professional satisfaction is at an all time low. Clearly, happiness is not solely a reflection of income. To regain a sense of happiness and fulfillment in their professional lives caregivers have to rediscover joy in their work. At a time when the pace of change makes the future unknowable, clinicians must make the journey and the destination the same.

The powerful forces of change mandate that healthcare providers separate substance from form.[6] Competition, changing expectations, and advancing technology are transforming what physicians do. Can physicians distinguish the essence of the role they play in society from those behaviors that are manifestations of how that role is currently being expressed? By analogy, transportation is an essential need. The vehicle changes over time. All of the forces for change cannot replace the intimacy of the doctor-patient relationship. Physicians have the privilege of being involved with people at their most intimate and vulnerable times. Many are willing to mortgage this privilege in deference to an economic model. The real challenge is to discover an economic model that preserves the opportunity to remain focused on the patient.

ACCEPTING RESPONSIBILITY FOR YOUR OWN FUTURE

As competition, technology, and consumerism transform the healthcare industry, many in the provider community have adopted the viewpoint of victims. They express feelings of anger, resentment, depression, and even hopelessness. In response, we suggest the only way to positively influence change is to engage it and proactively own your contribution to the present circumstances. It is not so much what happens as how you respond to what happens that is critical. You can control how you behave, and that is a way to assert a leadership influence.

If healthcare providers are to play a significant role in shaping the future of the healthcare industry, they must commit themselves to creating balanced accountability. As Donald Berwick has said proposed solutions must be balanced and acceptable to multiple stakeholders (Berwick 1997). Providers must commit to efficiency and respect the needs of the payers. They must propose solutions that are professionally and scientifically sound and be sensitive to meeting the needs of their patients and their families. And, if we are to restore a sense of joy to the provider community, the solutions must be acceptable to the human spirit.

The provider community must challenge itself to respond to the changing demands of society. Historical artifacts must be jettisoned as healthcare tries to remain integral with patients' changing needs. To endure, it must be adaptable and flexible and be able to reframe issues, and redefine and reinvent itself.

CONCLUSION

In this new world of technological advancement, innovation and creativity are more important than perfectibility. Dee Hock, founder of Visa, has likened creativity to the task of redecorating a room (Waldrop 1996). An endless variety of things could be put into the room, the challenge is deciding what to take out. Behavior is a reflection of underlying beliefs and attitudes. To change behavior, individuals must reevaluate those underlying beliefs and attitudes and take a look at their operating assumptions and evaluate whether those assumptions remain valid in the face of a significantly changing environment.

In healthcare, success cannot be achieved without the joint commitment of both organization and physicians to serving the needs of others. Individual success will be a derivative of collective success, and business success will derive from serving the needs of customers. This cannot occur without forming strong partnerships between healthcare organizations and those physicians who share the same vision and values. Failure to meet this challenge will be detrimental to patient and caregiver alike.

NOTES

1. Regina Herzlinger has written extensively on the impact of competition, consumerism, and technology on the healthcare industry (Herzlinger 1997). Her views are the basis for this discussion.
2. Our views on the impact of the new economy on healthcare are based on Kevin Kelly's book, *New Rules for the New Economy* (1998). The dynamics that are transforming other industries are clearly influencing healthcare. This book is a must read and forms the basis for much of the content in this chapter.
3. The impact of the forces deconstructing healthcare are visible everywhere. Evans and Wurster's book *Blown to Bits* clearly explains this dynamic and makes understandable the vulnerability of "full service

shops" (Evans and Wurster 2000). This phenomenon causes us to worry about the sustainability of the community-focused mission of not-for-profit healthcare organizations. The content on deconstruction is based on their discussion.

4. The compression of time and space explains one of the reasons why old-style top-down hierarchically controlled organizations cannot cope with the pace and magnitude of environmental change. *Edgeware* by Zimmerman, et al. provides a wonderful primer on complexity science and its applications to leadership and management in healthcare (Zimmerman and Plsek 1998).

5. Our views on meaning and purpose in work and on transformational relationships reflect the writings of Viktor Frankl (1985) and Stephen Covey (1994).

6. Our discussion on separating substance from form is adapted from Dee Hock (Waldrop 1996).

REFERENCES

Arbuckle, G. A. 1995. "Culture, Chaos, and Refounding." *Health Progress.* 76(2): 25–29, 48.

Beinhocker, E. D. 1999. "Robust Adaptive Strategies." *Sloan Management Review.* (Spring) 40(3).

Berwick, D. M. 1997. *The Ingredients of World-Class Health Care: Distinctive Characteristics of the Future Outstanding HealthCare Organizations.* Presented at VHA's Physician's Forum. Dallas, TX.

Collins, J., and J. Porras. 1997. *Built to Last: Successful Habits of Visionary Companies.* New York: Harper Collins.

Evans, P., and T. S. Wurster. 2000. *Blown to Bits: How the New Economics of Information Transforms Strategy.* Boston: Harvard Business School Press.

Frankel, V. E. 1984. *Man's Search for Meaning.* New York: Pocket Books.

Herzlinger, R. 1997. *Market-Driven Health Care: Who Wins Who Loses in the Transformation of America's Largest Service Industry.* Reading, MA: Addison-Wesley.

Kelly, K. 1999. *New Rules for the New Economy: 10 Radical Strategies for a Connected World.* New York: Penguin Group.

Mintzberg, H., and S. Glouberman. 1999. "Managing the Care of Health and the Cure of Disease, Part II: Integration." Unpublished paper.

Russell, P. 1998. *Waking Up in Time: Finding Inner Peace in Times of Accelerating Change.* Novato, CA: Origin Press.

Waldrop, M. M. 1996. "The Trillion-Dollar Vision of Dee Hock." *Fast Company* (Oct.) (5)75.

Wennberg, J. E., J. L. Freeman, and W. J. Culp. 1987. Are Hospital Services Rationed in New Haven or Over-Utilized in Boston? *Lancet* 23(1): 1185–9.

Wennberg, J. E. 1996. "The Dartmouth Atlas of Health Care in the United States." Chicago: American Hospital Association.

Zimmerman, B., and P. Plsek. 1998. *Edgeware.* Irving, TX: VHA, Inc.

Chapter Two

BARRIERS TO
SUCCESSFUL CHANGE

We don't see the world as it is but rather as we are.

The Talmud

A s the healthcare provider community struggles to respond to a dramatically changing environment, a number of organizational barriers and false assumptions predispose the community to failure. The inability to reduce or eliminate these barriers and the failure to clarify operating assumptions has limited adaptability and threatened the sustainability of healthcare organizations. In a similar manner, the failure to appreciate how the historical paradigms of medical practice no longer meet the needs of the society has precluded physician capacity to redefine and reimagine how the essence of the profession can be sustained within a model that better adapts to the needs of a changing environment.

ROADBLOCKS TO SUCCESSFUL ADAPTATION

Barriers within the provider community that markedly limit creativity and adaptability include:

- departmentalization,
- traditional physician approaches to patient care, and
- consensus management.

DEPARTMENTALIZATION

Almost all healthcare organizations are divided into discreet departments. Each department manager is held accountable to his or her departmental budget. Departmentalized budgeting is the easiest measurement to obtain and follow, and economic performance is historically the most important yardstick by which to assess performance. Each department manager is primarily evaluated and rewarded on the basis of his or her ability to manage within the allotted budget. While patient satisfaction, quality improvement initiatives, or other parameters may also be used to assess a manager's performance, performance in these areas is often difficult to measure.

Today, the progressively shrinking profit margins of healthcare organizations make adhering to budgeted performance even more heavily emphasized. This compartmentalizes the organization into vertical operating units in which each department seeks to optimize its own performance. It is a general principle of systems theory that for any system to operate at maximum efficiency no component of that system can operate at maximum efficiency. In effect, subsystem optimization suboptimizes the whole. Attempts to redesign work are compromised because no department wants to sacrifice its performance profile in deference to improving another.

Productivity indexing and departmental performance. Another barrier to change is using productivity indexing to judge departmental performance. Each department adopts a measure of productivity and then manages to optimize that measurement. Because manpower costs comprise the largest category of operating expense for healthcare organizations, attempts to hold departments accountable for units of production per full-time equivalent (FTE) employee are heavily emphasized.

Even holding meetings can become difficult because of departmental sensitivity to the loss of productivity consequent to the absence of a member who is away at the meeting. When ideas surface that would require one department altering its present approach to producing its unit of productivity, that department balks at the prospect of compromising its measured performance.

Although healthcare organizations are vertically organized into departments, patients use the healthcare system in a horizontal fashion that cuts across many individual departments. Managing this integrated system with collective accountability for the outcome is difficult because of the lack of any means to budget across the organizational structure.

Action-based accounting has been used to allocate indirect costs across departments in a service line situation. It allows healthcare organizations to reorganize workflow in a way that can integrate performance efficiency and assess effectiveness in a horizontal fashion across the organization (Gabram 1997). The following example demonstrates the application of action-based accounting. A large healthcare system owns a number of dialysis centers scattered throughout its service region. The centers are run in cooperation with a single group of nephrologists, and the system wants to sell the dialysis units because they no longer generate a profit. Two for-profit chains are competing to purchase the centers, which would continue to be managed in conjunction with the same group of doctors. Obviously, these for-profit chains believe they can generate a profit from managing dialysis centers. Considering that reimbursement is fixed by Medicare and that the physicians would be the same, how is it that the for-profits think they can create a profit? By not allocating to the centers all the areas of unrelated indirect cost that are traditionally allocated by hospitals, the chains calculate a profit. Profitability in this case is primarily a matter of accounting.

Productivity measurement systems can be used for benchmarking performance and assessing some parameters to maximize efficiency. However, this comparative assessment begins to lock organizations into the current way that the work is performed and does so in a manner that maintains the focus primarily on individual departmental functions and interferes with the ability to assess overall integrated performance. Thus, it blocks creativity and prevents the organization from adopting a horizontal view of organizational design. As organizations begin to deconstruct, it is imperative to reorganize along specific service lines. This process is inhibited by the current way that healthcare organizations budget and assess organizational performance.

TRADITIONAL PHYSICIAN APPROACHES TO CARE

Physicians are taught to serve as the patient's advocate.[1] Physicians have been trained in an era of insurance that has created the impression that financial resources are unlimited. Physicians behavior reflects the attitude that so long as no harm is done, the application of any ancillary service that might conceivably help their individual patient is justified, if not required. They do all that they can for the individual patient, seek not to differentiate the care provided on the basis of ability to pay, and feel ethically obligated to do so, thereby acting as the patient's advocate. As society has come to the realization that healthcare resources in fact are limited, they have turned to a managed care model as a means of creating financial accountability. Payers want physicians to make judgments that would support the greatest good for the greatest number. They want physicians to think not in terms of individual patients, but in terms of populations of patients. They want physicians to serve as the patients' advocates.

To most physicians, resource restrictions in the service of potential individual patient good is perceived as a compromise in quality of care. Therefore, if a managed cost approach to the allocation of healthcare resources is to be successful, this approach

26

must be shown not to compromise the clinical outcome of care, or it must demonstrate that the outcome is even enhanced by avoiding adverse consequences secondary to excessive care. Unfortunately, we collect very little outcome data, and most of it lacks comparability. Moreover, as David Eddy has said, the roles of serving as a patient's advocate are each attended by a separate and equally valid set of ethics, and no physician can simultaneously act in both capacities (Eddy 1998). This conflict poses an irresolvable dilemma for physicians who practice across these settings.

George Annas has characterized our society as being wasteful, technologically dependent, individualistic, and denying of death (Annas 1996). Given these characteristics, supported by our tort system, and patient perception of death as an optional event, it is no wonder that physicians have created a diagnostic and therapeutic model that is unaffordable. Moreover, a fee-for-service reimbursement model that economically rewards caregivers for what they do reinforces the entire dynamic — the more you do the more you are paid.

Physicians continue to act within the paradigms that they were taught in medical training. They have a loyalty to the fee-for-service model. Consistent with the target income principle (physicians will work to achieve a targeted level of income), most physicians have chosen to work harder to achieve their target. If reimbursement per unit of service decreases, then they do more units or shift their focus toward more profitable types of units to maintain their income. If the underlying belief is that medical care must be rendered one patient at a time, one patient to one doctor, the result is exhaustion, depression, and sadness. Time spent per patient decreases, intimacy is sacrificed, and consequently both the patient and the physician feel dissatisfied. Physicians must free themselves from the constraints of their historical beliefs and imagine new ways of delivering healthcare. For example, they might choose to create care models that generate revenue independent of their physical presence or that can deliver care to multiple patients simultaneously. Employing physician extenders (nonphysicians) could provide relief as would a willingness to capture discretionary spending for alternative healthcare services. Because the management of information is a critical new economy business, we can, for example, imagine physicians serving as the equivalent of an internet access provider for patients, helping to manage and interpret medical information for a monthly out-of-pocket fee. Unless physicians free themselves to imagine and dream, they will be prisoners of yesterday's models.

Physician extenders. Another barrier to change concerns the issue of the acceptability of physician extenders. Physicians have an acculturated bias that any activity performed by a nonphysician is inferior. Ample evidence exists to support the quality of care provided by nurse anesthetists and nurse midwives. Many of the problems faced by primary care providers can be managed by physician extenders with equivalent medical outcome, less cost, and higher levels of patient satisfaction. Nontraditional providers are often more successful than allopathic physicians in the management of chronic pain, back pain, headache, and a host of other chronic complaints. If physicians were to partner with physician extenders they could satisfy patients, access discretionary sources of revenue, create cash flow, and free up time for more complicated patient care issues that require more than a brief encounter sandwiched between two nonessential visits that are scheduled primarily to "pay the rent" (Reinertsen 1994).

CONSENSUS MANAGEMENT

Another block to successful adaptation by the provider community is the expectation that they manage for consensus agreement. This expectation exists in both the traditional hospital setting and within physician culture. Within the hospital setting an overriding concern prevails that all proposals be fair. Across-the-board budget cuts, proportional reductions in force, and standardization of nursing tasks across departments are just some behaviors that reflect this administrative imperative.

Physicians lack any frame of reference for how to work together away from the bedside. The only organizational model they have is the traditional medical staff structure. Anyone who has tried to conduct business at the medical staff level knows how frustrating and impossible a task it can be. In the absence of threat, little can be accomplished in a timely fashion. We have come to believe that the only thing that unites physicians is the mutual commitment to the preservation of individual physician prerogatives.

Physicians have no collective accountability. Within their expert culture, with some notable exceptions like rehabilitation and in-patient psychiatric services, the closest physicians could come, metaphorically speaking, to forming a team would be a golf team. The definition of success would be for each member to shoot the best individual score possible. Their contribution is to be as good an individual physician as they can be. If you want them to perform better, buy them some new clubs or give them golf lessons. Collective accountability beyond certain clinical settings is not a recognized need. Therefore, whenever they are asked to come together to develop collective judgments, they tend to favor the proposal that is the least objectionable to the most people. The overriding consideration is not to infringe on another physician's personal autonomy.

The innovation model. This behavior is in contrast with an approach based on the principles described by Everett Rogers (1995) in his dissemination of innovation model. In this model, populations are segmented into several types of members. A small group (2 1/2 percent), called innovators, like novelty and seek new ideas. Their frame of reference is external to their peer group that generally cannot discern if the innovators are ingenious, crazy, or both. For this reason innovators do not influence the mainstream. The next group, termed early adopters (13 1/2 percent), is the key to disseminating change. This group is open to new ideas and willing to experiment in search of potential application. They are distinguished from the innovators by being legitimate members of the larger group and therefore able to influence them. The next group, the early majority (33 1/3 percent), has a local frame of reference. They distrust ideas imported from outside. They are, however, influenced by observing the behavior of the early adopters.

Once members of the early majority can observe new ideas that are successfully incorporated into changing local behaviors by the early adopters, they begin to copy these changes and adoption of the changes becomes unstoppable. Given this model, as Don Berwick has advised, one can lead for change by exposing early adopters to selected new ideas. Since all truly new ideas are imported, this requires sending early adopters "out of town" for an opportunity to discover innovations. By allowing the early adopters to experiment with these innovations and to reinvent them locally to improve the fit and legitimize them, one can create an opportunity for the early majority to observe the changes and judge their adoptability (Berwick 1996). Leading and managing change using this pull strategy is far more effective than pushing from behind in an attempt to manage for consensus.

Managing for consensus cannot be effective in the absence of a strong external threat to the entire group. All groups act in defense of the status quo. Whenever those who would articulate for change try to persuade an entire group of the rectitude of their proposal, they encounter resistance (O'Toole 1995). Inevitably, the desire to manage for consensus agreement results in no significant change. When a group is hiking, if the dominant intention is to stay together (consensus management), the slowest walker determines the speed of the group. The accelerating pace of change demands enhanced adaptability, and managing for consensus significantly compromises innovation. A politically riskier but more effective approach focuses efforts on the early adopters and creates change with pull rather than push strategies. The metaphor of a slinky toy emphasizes this strategic approach. Creating small successes that are measurable, visible, and meaningful generates positive momentum and an atmosphere of trust, hope, and optimism that the group can act on to create its own future. Small successes on the part of early adopters serve to pull the group toward new behaviors.

FALSE ASSUMPTIONS

Other barriers to successful adaptation are false assumptions. Some of these false assumptions include the following:

- a strong primary care physician base is necessary,
- physicians are data driven,
- individuals lack motivation to achieve high levels of performance,
- focusing on improving employee job satisfaction is important; and
- biases that underlie attempts to create new physician-organization relationships.

BUILDING A STRONG PRIMARY CARE BASE

A strong primary care base is generally believed to be essential for the success of hospital-based healthcare organizations. In many areas of the country, hospitals and health systems have purchased the practices of primary care physicians throughout their service region. Others have sought to hire primary care physicians directly. The rationale is to provide referrals to the medical specialists who apply their technical expertise in conjunction with the hospital and generate most of the profit. Therefore, they want to own or control a large feeder base of primary care doctors. A desire to control the medical continuum of care or the intent to participate in a primary care/gatekeeper model of capitation may also drive this strategy. To date, the majority of hospital or health system–owned physician practices are not profitable.

However, the notion really does not make sense. When a patient calls to make an appointment to see a primary care physician, many of those who call actually do not need to see anyone. They want information, reassurance, or direction. Other patients have either self-limited or imagined disease, and often a physician extender can see them and create an equivalent medical outcome for less cost with a higher level of service satisfaction. A few need to proceed directly to the emergency room, and others, especially those with dermatologic or endocrine symptoms, are seen more efficiently and effectively through direct referral to the appropriate specialist.

In fact, demand management programs are beginning to disintermediate primary care physicians from this role in the doctor-patient relationship. Information and advice are provided through access to a triage nurse or other intermediary, thereby bypassing the additional and often unnecessary cost of seeing the primary care physician. Imagine the impact on primary care physicians if nurse practitioners or pharmacists were authorized to write prescriptions, or if patients could purchase pharmaceuticals over-the-counter as is the case in many countries. A concern exists for the long-term viability of family practice physicians who continue to practice in urban areas. If the above dynamic is in fact correct, the progressive cost constraints in healthcare will act to devalue family practitioners to the economic level of the lowest cost physician extender.

Although primary care physicians may have a limited future in their current capacity, they have an unlimited value in a very different role—managing patient information and helping patients navigate the complexities of a world where there is an overload of information. Additional strategies that could serve to sustain the practice of primary care physicians would be to expand their practices to include physician extenders with whom they would not compete and to whom they would defer routine functions while they seek to move up-market by utilizing new technologies that allow them to do in their office setting what used to be performed by specialists in more expensive and inconvenient settings[2] (Christensen 1997).

PHYSICIANS ARE DATA DRIVEN

People assume that physicians are data driven. It is widely believed that competitive physicians, when presented with data demonstrating that their performance differs from their peers, will act to self-correct their behavior to bring their performance in line with others. This approach to the use of data may create some level of compliance when the physician is strongly motivated by either reward or threat, but it almost never creates commitment to or enrollment in the new behavior.

Physicians and perfection. Physicians must believe that what they do in caring for patients is perfect. Patients, society, the tort system, and their own cultural expectations demand it. If physicians believe that what they are doing is perfect, proposals to change what they are doing is interpreted as compromising the quality of care, usually for someone else's economic gain. Moreover, doing less is additionally perceived as increasing both risk of litigation and patient dissatisfaction. Since change is initially clumsy, with no perceived need to change, why do it?

Physicians are exposed to data in one of two ways, either in support of scientific discovery or for purposes of peer review. In the former, the gold standard is the single variable, prospective, randomized, double-blinded trial with a significant N and P value.

Clinical data in the healthcare setting are never that precise. Demanding the application of tests of statistical significance to the data is meaningless. However, when this level of significance cannot be substantiated, the individualistic and scientific-minded physician denies any meaning to the data and continues behaving as before. Physicians must appreciate that the real utility of healthcare data is to generate dialog around the possible implications of the data and to generate higher-level questions. Different approaches cannot all be best.

Applying a decision tree that judges proposals in the following order of priority is useful: (1) Is the proposed change more or equally effective? (2) Is it equally safe or safer? and (3) If the first two conditions are satisfied, is it less costly? In this way, dialog among peers focusing on variations in approaches to diagnosis and therapy becomes an avenue for discovery and improvement. Of course, measurements must be in place to guide judgment. The attempt to apply evidence-based medical guidelines is one example of how this dynamic can be supported.

Peer review. Peer review has emerged in a context of a quality assurance model. Indicator flags cause certain charts to "fall out" for peer review to ensure that the clinical quality of care rendered meets minimal standards of acceptability. The review is a measurement for judgment, and almost universally despised by both those reviewing and those being reviewed. Peer review is viewed as an attempt to justify the care given or to rationalize an adverse outcome. It lacks the mind-set of quality improvement where measurement is applied for improvement, not judgment. Because of the judgmental nature of the peer review process, physicians will discredit data that challenge the current level of their performance. Failing that, they will claim that their patients are in some way unique and thereby justify the data. Finally, if the above two responses fail to stall initiatives that would seek to change their behavior, they will act out in ways that simulate "shooting the messenger."

Notably, physicians are often correct in their objections. The data are far from perfect, the patient population often is significantly different, and sometimes interventions that are primarily financially motivated do justify assassinating the messenger. The process of peer review, that is, measurement for judgment, should remain in the domain of credentialing and privileging and not be merged with performance improvement initiatives. Quality improvement seeks to focus on process improvement, enhancing the aggregate quality of care provided, and making good care better. Frustratingly, no matter how these two different activities are performed, physicians constantly revert to a defensive mind-set. It is a reflection of a culture that demands perfection and assigns accountability to the individual clinician. Merging these two distinctive activities makes it all the harder to move past a culture of blame toward one of improvement.

Physicians require data to change behavior. Brent James[3] at Intermountain Health Care makes the following point: To change physician behavior in a way that creates a commitment to or enrollment in a new behavior requires that the data presented address the level of the underlying belief that justifies the current behavior (James 1999). For example, one urologist had his patients in the hospital almost two days longer than his peers when performing a transurethral resection of the prostate gland. Despite the data, his behavior remained unchanged. When challenged, he replied that his patients were hospitalized longer because they were receiving better care. He was trained that to remove a bladder catheter before the patient's urine was clear of all visible signs of blood was to increase the risk that the patient would require recatheterization to relieve clot obstruction of the bladder. When data were collected that demonstrated that his peer's patients did not require more frequent recatheterizations despite having their catheters removed two days earlier, he willingly changed his behavior. The data addressed the underlying belief. Until the data demonstrated objectively that the new behavior did not compromise quality of care, the physician re-fused to change his behavior for what he believed to be legitimate reasons.

As scientists, physicians are more easily influenced by data than anecdote. However, their clinical behavior is not solely depend-ent on knowledge. If it were, continuing medical education and the publication of evidence-based guidelines of care would have a significant impact on the details of care provided. In fact, physi-cians tend to practice the medicine they were taught in training and only change when they personally become dissatisfied with the outcome of the care it generates. As long as what they are do-ing appears to be working, they will continue to do the familiar rather than change. And unless the data presented to the contrary address the level of the belief that justifies the current behavior, the data will be denied.

A change in mind-set is required. Physicians need to adopt an at-titude of seeing measurement for improvement and not judg-ment.[4] They need to again become curious and seek to make the good better. Moreover, they need to appreciate that efficiency and effectiveness are opposite sides of the same coin. The right per-son, doing the right thing, in the right way, at the right time, and in the right place will create the best outcome for the least cost. Those parameters must be defined.

Another issue relating to physicians and data reflects the ori-gin of most healthcare data. These data are predominantly gen-erated in service of financial ends. When reconstituted to serve clinical purposes, they fail to reflect clinical context and become summarily rejected by clinicians. This unmasks a very real para-dox. When healthcare organizations approach physicians about controlling the cost of care, physicians become suspicious and distrustful. On the other hand, failure to elicit physician account-ability for the economic outcomes of care will serve to threaten the organization's solvency. Healthcare providers must begin col-lecting data that balance all of the relevant outcomes of the care provided. In addition to financial outcome this should include measures of medical outcome, patient satisfaction with how they experienced the care, and caregiver pride in how that care was rendered.

INDIVIDUALS LACK MOTIVATION

All individuals are 100 percent motivated 100 percent of the time. The challenge is to direct that motivation. Charles Dwyer proposes that you can get anyone to do anything anytime if you are willing to take the risk and pay the price.[5] Organizations are a collection of individuals who show up each day to maximize what they personally value. Specific behaviors will only be adopted if an offer is made that creates the *perception* that adopting the behavior they seek will serve to enhance what it is that *they* personally *value* (Dwyer 1992).

The emphasized words are very critical. It is about perception and not logic. It is all about packaging. Identifying what the individual values is important because the proposal must promise to enhance that value. If the individual still refuses to change, you should respond by assessing the following five important parameters.

- Does the person have the capacity to do what is asked?
- Is the promise probable?
- Can you be trusted?
- What is the cost of the new behavior?
- What is the risk?

Most importantly, accept personal responsibility for not structuring the offer properly. If the person does not have the capacity to do what is asked can you provide them with the opportunity, skills, and/or knowledge to be able to do so. Present the data that support the validity of the quid pro quo that is proposed. If they do what is asked, how likely are the anticipated results to occur?

37

Assess the perception of the possibility of this quid pro quo being realized. This is primarily a matter of trust. If they perform as requested and the anticipated results ensue, can you be trusted to pay off? What can you do to enhance their perception of your trustworthiness?

Individuals overestimate the cost of change. All individuals will overestimate the personal cost to changing. This cost may be in the form of effort, time, or money. To positively influence this judgment, you must decrease perception of the cost. Salespersons often use this approach. For example, they might ask if you would like to purchase their product or service for a given amount per year. If you say no, the salesperson will show you how the total cost per day becomes "easily affordable," $365.00 per year is a lot of money, but $1.00 per day is very doable.

Risk involved in change. All people will overestimate the personal risk of change. To overcome this barrier, you have to change their perception of the amount of risk. This may be accomplished through spreading out the risk and showing how others are participating in the new behavior. This is especially effective when the willing participants have a strong reputation. Pharmaceutical salespersons often invoke this approach when trying to influence physicians. They reference local specialists as already utilizing a new drug, creating the impression of its proven worth. Not being the first and or only person to adopt a new behavior is comforting and reassuring.

Physicians are not generic in the way they prioritize their personal values. Their chosen area of practice often reflects their hierarchy of values. Primary care physicians generally choose that specialty because relationships are of major importance to them. In contrast, radiologists tend to prefer science and technology to relationships. Pathologists and many internists are attracted to the more intellectual challenges of diagnosis. Surgeons are active and enjoy the immediate rewards of "fixing things." Pediatricians and family practice physicians are "warm and fuzzy" individuals who are responsive to approaches that are inclusive, sensitive, and preserving of relationships. Neurosurgeons and cardiovascular surgeons want to be in control and get to the point, make a decision, move on, and "let the chips fall where they may." These are obvious generalizations, but various medical staff departments do tend to reflect a characteristic personality. What appeals to and motivates one group is likely to be different from what influences another. Appreciating that individual physicians prioritize values differently allows for the opportunity to create a relevant context and the ability to make appealing offers.

THE MYTH OF EMPLOYEE SATISFACTION

The importance of managing to continually enhance employee satisfaction is another false assumption (Atchison 1999). An emphasis on employee satisfaction surveys are an attempt to respond to the growing sense of dissatisfaction that is affecting healthcare professionals. Administrators want to respond to the increasing unhappiness and improve morale by identifying and improving areas that become evident through these survey results. Excellent service quality is an idea that is catching on in healthcare organizations, and unhappy employees are finding it difficult to provide a cheerful, service-oriented environment. The notion that enhancing employee satisfaction will improve performance is a myth. What contributes to employee retention and performance is pride in the workplace, and pride comes from finding meaning and purpose in work. It results from factors like respect, competence, collegiality, and a sense of shared purpose in doing something that matters.

Continually seeking to satisfy employees serves to reinforce a mind-set of entitlement and to raise the bar of expectations. Employees will never be totally satisfied. Employers can always do more to provide a more satisfying environment. Issues of safety, cleanliness, and other aspects of a comfortable environment are important to morale, but only to a point. Paying attention to those factors that contribute to employee pride is important. While minimum levels of parameters exist for accepting employment, once those minimums are met, pride in performance, recognition, appreciation, and the integration of shared purpose that should be the focus of attention.

BIASES ABOUT FORMING NEW PHYSICIAN-ORGANIZATION RELATIONSHIPS

Significant prejudices attend current attempts to create physician-organizational partnerships. Almost all of the dialog has been about governance and economics. Initial intentions have focused on acquiring the arbitrage profits that were seen as accruing to managed care companies, and almost all of the expressed views have been in the first person: This is what I want. This is what we need.

An emphasis on governance reflects the deep-seated distrust that exists between physicians and administration. Administration and its board want to protect their capital investment from the "greediness" of physicians, who in turn fear being controlled by the organization. Within the limits of legal requirements, governance has approximated 50-50 or 51-49, and physician membership on the new entity governing board has been representational. The underlying message is that organizations and physicians do not trust each other, and that the physicians do not trust each other either. Physicians elected to the boards are often not the most qualified, but rather those who will look out for the perceived interests of their specific specialty peers. Similarly, almost all ventures have been inclusive, because it has been thought too politically risky to be selective.

Those physicians best prepared to lead their colleagues into the world of the new economy are often not among the group of physicians who are most respected by their colleagues. Physicians tend to respect those peers who are clinically outstanding. This is in keeping with their experiences in medical training in which those with the most prestige were the ones most clinically competent. Paradoxically, those physicians who best understand the economic forces that are transforming healthcare are often those least vested in the historical paradigms, sometimes because they have not been successful working within those paradigms. Although they may be best positioned to lead these new efforts, they lack their colleagues' respect and so are rejected in part on that basis.

Once physicians and administrators agree to start a business relationship, both parties immediately seek to create structure with the dominant focus initially on governance issues. Little time is spent on clarifying the what and why of the relationship; what it will look like, why they are coming together, and what metric will define success. The parties do not discuss and prioritize collective values. They do not imagine multiple potential futures and ask themselves how they will respond to various eventualities. These discussions would bring to life how those collective values would serve as a compass to guide future decision making and clarify the purpose of the relationship.

Both clinicians and healthcare organizations behave as though patients are commodities and see them as pawns in a game of chess played against payers and insurers. Whereas the organization focuses on controlling distribution channels and creating geographic presence to ensure long-term survival, physicians seek to protect their short-term income and autonomy and to capture income through controlling ancillary services. For each group, the assumption that structure will create function is flawed. Rarely is an infrastructure in place to help manage care or risk.

Somehow providers presume that because they are in the business of taking care of patients, efficient and effective results will automatically be forthcoming. The insurance and administrative functions are an incidental nuisance and an excuse for the organizations that perform those functions to just skim profits off the top. Greed in pursuit of arbitrage profits has driven the providers' desire to secure risk contracts well in advance of their ability to manage the risk. In addition, the number of plan enrollees has often been small and the resulting actuarial risk has not been supportable and clearly not within the control of the providers. In effect, providers have underestimated the complexities of the insurance business.

CONCLUSION

Unless the provider community can overcome some of the barriers and false operating assumptions that inhibit innovative and creative responses to the changing demands of society, it will remove itself from the opportunity to successfully coauthor its own future. Rather it will remain locked in the mind-set of a victim forced to reluctantly respond in a reactive manner to externally imposed demands. Healthcare is experiencing its own form of paradigm paralysis, refusing to acknowledge the legitimacy of the expectations of its customers. As with all paradigm shifts, the power base and economic rewards will change, and control will pass to those who can successfully adapt.

Organizations must restructure. Deciding what to measure, actively measuring it, and providing real-time feedback of that measurement to those who need to access that information is a critical first step. Measurement is its own self-fulfilling prophecy. Once you decide to measure something change is created in the direction intended. Currently, the focus of measurement is locked into financial performance as judged by departmentalized budgeting and productivity indexing. Indeed, within healthcare organizations the most easily measured parameters are financial, and therefore the fiscal bottom line becomes the essential purpose of the organization by default.

A budgeting process that breaks the organization into discreet departments prevents a systems perspective of work and misaligns the organization. Productivity measures that guide components toward optimizing their piece of the work promote withholding of information and suboptimizing the whole in deference to the performance profile of individual parts. More importantly, it limits creativity and reinforces business as usual. Incentives must be aligned. Effective teamwork integrates expectations and accountabilities across the team. In addition, for meaningful change to occur within organizations the historical power and reward systems must be altered. This naturally meets resistance from those who benefit from the status quo. Aligning the organization is the responsibility of senior administration. This is no easy task. Entitlements, human resource policies, traditional unionism, and myriad other forces resist changes that threaten the security of individual workers. Only a powerful unifying vision and the creation of a culture around shared goals and values can accomplish this endeavor.

Physicians must free themselves from the paradigm paralysis of traditional medical practice. This requires the ability to separate substance from form, purpose from mission. The medical profession works within the context of the larger society of which it is a part. The expectations of that society are changing. If mission is the vestment that clothes purpose, then society is asking for a change of clothes. The essence of the profession and the role it plays in society cannot change, but the form in which that essence is made manifest must change. Physicians must put on a new wardrobe in response to the changing season. All four points on the value compass must be served. It is no longer sufficient to defend medical quality through attestation. Outcomes must be measured. Also, physicians can no longer point to a satisfactory medical outcome as the soul justification for how they created that outcome. They must become additionally accountable for the economic outcomes of that care, the quality of how the patient and his or her family experienced that care, and the spiritual context in which caregivers and patients interact. Don Berwick has challenged the healthcare industry to acknowledge that units of production are not the fundamental business of healthcare, rather the relationship of caregiver to patient. "We are guests in their lives, not hosts in our organization." We must adopt a mind-set of measurement for improvement and not measurement for judgment (Berwick 1999).

NOTES

1. David Eddy has described the ethical dilemma that physicians face when they are asked to serve simultaneously as the ombudsman for an individual patient and as an agent for the collective good of society. He refers to this as the problem of an apostrophe. I heard him offer this construct at a presentation sponsored by VHA (Eddy 1998).
2. Clayton Christensen's book, *The Innovator's Dilemma*, characterizes the challenges to today's successful healthcare organizations. The paradigm is shifting and organizations will fail not because they are poorly managed, but precisely because they are well managed. He distinguishes disruptive technologies that transform industries from sustaining technologies that serve to move mainstream businesses further up-market. The consequences of technological advances are for the site of service to move closer to the customer and for the provider of that service to be progressively less well trained. The result is lower cost and more convenience and an expansion of markets to those segments that previously could not afford the product or service (Christensen 1997).
3. Brent James, a surgeon at Intermountain Health Care in Utah, has vast experience with clinical process improvement. James observes that commitment to or enrollment in new behaviors requires the presentation of supporting data that address the level of the belief that justifies the current behavior. Brent is at the pinnacle of the clinical quality improvement movement, and any articles that he has authored are insightful accounts.
4. Measurement for improvement is a phrase I have heard Don Berwick use. At an annual address to the Institute for Healthcare Improvement he voiced the opinion that in order for physicians to regain a position of influence in the evolving healthcare system, they

must propose solutions that are balanced and address the needs of payers, science, customer/family, and the human spirit (Berwick 1999).

5. Chuck Dwyer is a professor at the Wharton School of Business and a presenter for the American College of Physician Executives in its Physicians in Management seminar series. This concept was part of his content area in that series.

REFERENCES

Annas, G. I. 1996. "Toward an Ecology of Health Beyond the Military and Market Metaphors." *Health Forum* 39(3): 30–34.

Atchison, T. A.. 1999. "The Myths of Employee Satisfaction." *Healthcare Executive* 14(2): 18–23.

Berwick, D. M. 1996. "Sauerkraut, Sobriety and The Spread of Change." Presented to the Eightieth Annual National Forum on Quality Improvement in Health Care. New Orleans, LA.

Berwick, D. M. 1999. Keynote address at the meeting of the Institute for Healthcare Improvement. New Orleans, LA.

Christensen, C. 1997. *The Innovator's Dilemma*. Boston: Harvard Business School Press.

Dwyer, C. E. 1992. *The Shifting Sources of Power and Influence*. Tampa, FL: American College of Physician Executives.

Eddy, D. 1998. Presentation made at a meeting of VHA's Physician Leadership Council. Dallas, TX.

Gabram, S. G., R. A. Mendola, J. Rozenfeld, and R. L. Gamelli. 1997. "Why Activity Based Accounting Works." *Physician Executive* 26(6): 31–37.

O'Toole, J. 1995. *Leading Change: Overcoming the Ideology of Comfort and the Tyranny of Custom*. San Francisco: Jossey-Bass.

Reinersten, J. L. 1994. "Leading Clinical Quality Improvement: The Tyranny of Piecework, Political and Practical Milestones." *Health Forum* 37(4): 18–21, 23–4.

Rogers, E. M. 1995. *Diffusions of Innovations*. New York: Free Press.

Chapter Three

PERCEPTION AND CHANGE

When one door closes, another opens; but we often look so long and so regretfully upon the closed door that wo do not see the one which has opened for us.

Alexander Graham Bell

Take your brain out and jump on it—it gets all caked up.

Mark Twain

T HE WAY WE, as human beings, view the world controls our thoughts, feelings, and behavior. At birth we arrive with a genetically determined potential to evolve through a predictable developmental series. These developmental phases cannot be altered. However, the most important aspect of development is our interaction with the environment.

Socialization is the process that imprints our perceptions of the world. Life experiences are affected to a large degree by our genetic predisposition — especially in the early years. The longer we live and the more experiences we have determines the way we view the world. Our biases, prejudices, values, and beliefs are carved deeply into our psyches. All behaviors are a function of the genetic package we receive at conception and the way this

47

genetic package is formed and shaped through multiple experiences with life. Life experiences are the socialization process that determines how we view the world and how we behave. These interactions with the environment predetermine perceptual responses.

How socialization creates perceptual biases and how these perceptions control behaviors unlock the mysteries of the change management process. The one fact that underlies all perceptual dynamics is that, "All humans are 100 percent correct 100 percent of the time—from their point of view." This fundamental principal is the key to understanding organizational dynamics and managing change. This chapter will explain the triggers and filters that control perception; examine decision models based on perceptual bias; present basic lessons of perception; and discuss how perception and change management intertwine.

STIMULUS CONTROL

All behaviors are sandwiched between two variables: antecedent conditions and consequences. An antecedent condition is any condition or event that stimulates (i.e., triggers a predictable cluster of responses). One theoretical model of human behavior suggests that antecedent stimuli control most behaviors.

We have learned that certain stimuli or symbols mean that certain behaviors are more appropriate. For example, when we enter a church, the symbolic nature of the surroundings directs our subconscious control mechanisms to produce a cluster of behaviors that are adaptable to the church environment (e.g., silence, kneeling, praying, listening). A contrary example would be attending a professional basketball game. The stadium will elicit a pattern of behaviors that is different in many respects from the pattern presented in the church setting. These behavioral triggers are unconscious and are created over time as a function of our developmental, social experiences. Different symbols have more or less power to control behavior. The frequency and quality of our relationship to that stimulus determine the amount of control any stimulus possesses. In short we are the sum of our experiences, our history creates our current perceptual reality. Our historical relationship to the stimulus potential of all events we experience is a learned relationship.

The fact that these relationships are learned means that they can be unlearned, weakened, strengthened, and/or replaced. The problem that arises when thinking about changing behavior is how to determine the strength of the bond between the stimulus and the response (S–R). The nature of the S–R bond is unconscious. Much of the time we do not know what is controlling our response pattern. Only through watching behaviors over a period of time can the bond between stimulus and behavior be identified.

TRIGGERS

Triggers are symbols that reliably elicit predictable clusters of behaviors. A common example of a trigger is a traffic light. Driving a car is a great deal safer when everyone on the road stops for a red light, proceeds on a green light, and is cautious on approaching a yellow light. The color of the light subconsciously triggers these responses because of the social conditioning process that begins very early in our lives.

Triggers involving healthcare. In healthcare academic credentials, professional licenses, titles, office location, and length of service are just some of the more potent symbols that control (trigger) predictable responses. Imagine the response possibilities upon meeting a 30-year-old women for the first time who says she works in healthcare. One immediate, and fairly predictable, response might be the expectation that she is a nurse. When she tells you she is a physician, a new response cluster emerges. When she tells you she is the chief cardiac surgeon, yet another response cluster results. Finally, she tells you that she is fed up with the way

49

healthcare has changed and is leaving her practice to spend time with her children and garden. Another set of responses may occur. Each one of our responses is controlled by our perception, biases, and beliefs. Our historical relationship with gender, age, race, sexual preference, titles, and personal values significantly affects how we view a situation. Therefore, how we behave is a function of our history with the symbol and the consistency or inconsistency of the current situation. Too many changes in the symbols that have controlled our behavior can cause very serious adjustment reactions. We do not know what to do or how to behave.

The dynamics between triggers and behavior. The relationship between symbols and the behaviors they trigger become especially important in mergers, large reorganizations, and constant change. For example mergers usually result in a new name for the organization. In the last several years, some these new names seem to have been created through the random selection of vowels and consonants or by dropping Scrabble letters onto a table. What was St. Elsewhere Hospital and Community General Hospital is now one corporation—Intergalactic Health System. Staff and community members will likely continue to call one facility "St. E's" and the other "Community." The lesson to managing change during and after a merger is to never underestimate the historical relationship humans have with symbols, or, in this case, names. The same lesson holds true for large-scale reorganizations and continuous change in which job titles are modified, offices are moved, and roles and responsibilities are altered. People learn a specific cluster of behaviors associated with their own and their colleagues' titles and roles. Significant changes in these potent symbols confuse the trigger response, sometimes to the point of incapacity to perform. Changing symbols always causes some pause and many times regression. Effective change management plans must anticipate and understand the importance of symbols and how they trigger behavior.

FILTERS

Filters are like triggers in that they control behavior and are a function of our socialization process, but dynamically the two are very different. Triggers are symbols that predictably stimulate behavior. Filters are cognitive processes wherein we assess a universe of data and select from the totality of these data elements that data point which most reinforces what we believe in the first place. Humans subconsciously select evidence that supports their predispositions. Humans want to be right. Therefore, we begin each interaction with specific, subconscious biases (i.e., our perception of the truth). We systematically discount any points of view that run counter to our truth and exaggerate the value and validity of any data that support our beliefs. This cognitive phenomenon is sometimes to referred to as a "self-fulfilling prophecy" or the Pygmalion effect.

Filters may explain resistance to change. Filters explain much of an individual's or a group's resistance to change. When an individual decides that a merger is just an economic manipulation that has no positive effect on quality, that person will discount any quality improvement efforts and point out all economic issues. If a CEO believes that physicians are only motivated by money, the CEO will ignore all of the committee work, extra office work, and staff training that occur far more often than discussions about compensation.

Human biases are learned; therefore, they can be unlearned. However, the amount of evidence needed to overcome a predisposition is overwhelming. Replacing incorrect or dysfunctional perceptions (filters) with notions that are supported by current reality is difficult, requires many contraindicative experiences, and takes a long time.

The leadership lesson to altering filters comes down to one word—*results*. No amount of talking will convince someone that his or her view of the world is wrong. Only hard, behaviorally specific evidence will weaken and ultimately modify a strongly held bias. The *only* remedy to skepticism are *results* that are different from the skeptic's bias. Real change is in the doing—not the talking.

DECISION MODELS

Our social history determines the way we make decisions. Each of us began as a cluster of genetically designed potential. Our interactions with the environment systematically shaped our behavior within genetic limits. The way we make and communicate decisions is based on our triggers and filters. Some patterns of decision making can be generalized. The way physicians make decisions is different from the way executives and lawyers make them. Physicians are conditioned to view a large amount of data and come to a conclusion (i.e., a diagnosis). For example, the letter "V" is broad at the top and quickly comes to a point. This describes the decision model of physicians. Attorneys, on the other hand, take a data point and, through the Socratic method, expand the point to a vast number of difficult-to-answer questions. Think of an upside down V. The executive's decision model differs from both of these groups. Executives look at the data and try to deduce some "what ifs." Their scenario-building cognitive motif can be displayed by two "WW's." The multiple points at the bottom represent options based on the data presented. When these diverse decision models are combined with the dynamics of triggers and filters, there is little wonder why meetings among doctors, lawyers, and executives can be frustrating for all parties.

LESSONS OF PERCEIVED REALITY

The evidence that our perception controls how we behave is very compelling. Triggers, filters, and decision models show that our reality is determined by our history within specific social structures. Knowledge of how perception controls reality is very useful

Figure 3.1   Always Start Discussions About Change at the Point of Greatest Agreement

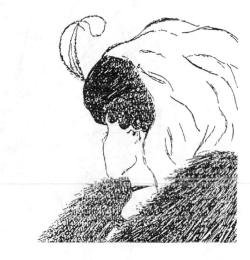

in change management interventions. The following perceptual illusions offer several lessons for leaders trying to manage change with physicians and other healthcare professionals.

Leadership Lesson: Always start discussions about change at the point of greatest agreement.

The illusion in Figure 3.1 is of a woman. Depending on how the figure is viewed, it is either an old woman or a young woman. "All humans are 100 percent correct, 100 percent of the time — from their point of view." Therefore, whenever two or more groups view a situation differently, the challenge for leadership is to accept all beliefs as valid and try to find some common ground within the diversity of thoughts. Too often people begin discussing change goals by identifying the points of greatest

Figure 3.2   Think Small, Move Fast, and Fix the Fixable

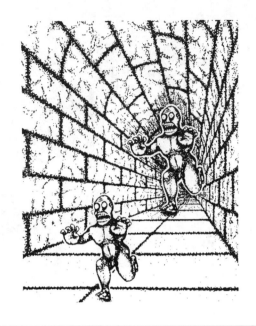

disagreement. This creates a polemic atmosphere wherein compromise or collaboration cannot exist.

Leadership Lesson: Think small, move fast, and fix the fixable.

The two objects in Figure 3.2 are exactly the same height. The figure in the back looks larger because of the background environment. In our multitask and stressful environment, we sometimes cluster problems. The result of this clustering process is a background of difficulties that are perceived to be much greater than any one problem individually. The key to change management is to separate the problems into manageable bits and deal with each one individually.

Figure 3.3   Always Start a Change Process with a Clear
Understanding of What Success Looks Like

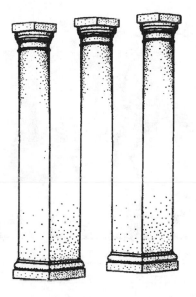

Leadership Lesson: Always start a change process with a clear understanding of what success looks like.

In any change management process a critical factor is the definition of success. Change management discussions often are consumed with clarification and analyses of what is wrong. While these discussions can be informative, they in no way describe the desirable outcome. A poignant question that must dominant the change leader's thought process is, "Would we recognize success if we tripped over it?" The columns illusion in Figure 3.3 represents the modus operandi of many change attempts. The dialog is passionate about the fact that the columns are broken and need to be fixed; however, no one clarifies whether the problem

Figure 3.4   The Ideal Situation Is to Create a Balance Between the Tangibles and Intangibles

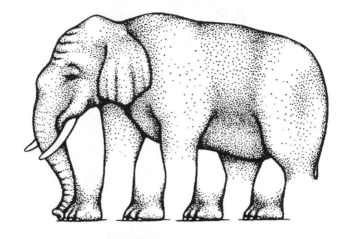

is solved when we build round or square columns. Too often energy is used to clarify the problem rather than the successful outcome. Effective change leaders call this process creating a shared vision.

Leadership Lesson: The ideal situation is to create a balance between the tangibles and the intangibles.

The illusion in Figure 3.4 is a metaphor for all organizational change. The head and body of the elephant represent the organization's strategic and financial plans. The legs represent the people who need to implement the plans. "Alignment" is one of the most important words in change management. Leaders understand that change is easy when the people and the plans are aligned. Likewise, no good can result when the desires of the people and the goals of the organization are misaligned. This chapter began with a discussion about the tangibles and the intangibles. The elephant illusion is also a description of the relationship between these two domains. Plans typically do not fail because they were badly constructed. They fail because the intangibles were not aligned with the tangibles.

PHYSICIAN FACTORS AND CHANGE MANAGEMENT

The way we view the world is a function of our socialization process. Physicians as a group have been socialized according to some consistent educational and interpersonal experiences. For example, competition for grades begins at a very early age. Competitive behavior is considered desirable. Achievement of number one status in class is a clear goal. Selection to a top university is critical. The quality of the resident match defines the degree of success. Throughout this long process of becoming a physician, the social dynamic tends to develop a degree of narcissism. The result of this process of competition, excellence, and narcissism is an individual who has powerful triggers and filters as well as a perceptual reality that is foreign to other professionals in the healthcare environment. The sum of these dynamics and the potential conflicts with other staff in the healthcare setting is covered in the next chapter under Expert Culture. However, some dominant triggers, filters, and perceptual realities deserve consideration.

PHYSICIAN TRIGGERS AND FILTERS

Triggers are symbols. The letters and titles after one's name, such as M.D., FACP, Chief of Cardiovascular Surgery, or other symbols such as the white coat, the stethoscope, even body language produce predictable responses in those who interact with these symbols. Traditionally, the symbol M.D. resulted in respectful deferment to the physician's decisions. The physician's body language might even trigger a bit of fear that may eliminate dialog about other options. The totality of symbols that are manifest by physicians is huge and controls a great deal of behavior because of the trigger phenomenon.

Filters help explain why change is unusually difficult for physicians. Filters are biases and prejudices that cause an individual to discount any data that runs counter to her beliefs and to exaggerate the value of any data that supports her initial presumptions. Some of the most common filters or assumptions associated with physicians are:

- Physicians are only interested in money.
- Working with physicians is like herding cats.
- Physicians view administration as "the suits."
- Physicians are not interested in the greater good provided by the health system.

Each of these biases serves as a filter to perceptions that would otherwise promote partnerships.

Physicians' filters are often equally potent barriers to cooperation. Physicians may begin a dialog with such a firm position that reasonable alternatives or even slight modifications in their position are filtered as "anti-physician" behavior. For example, physicians may view the executive team as "the suits" who do nothing but go from meeting to meeting. They may consider any denied capital request as further deterioration of quality or that creating community-based clinics are a way for the healthcare system to compete directly with their practices.

Of course, triggers and filters can be positive in the management of change. The first challenge is to understand perceptual controls. Do executives view physicians as competitors? Is the executive physician friendly or physician hostile? Has the executive ever discounted a physician's idea because the idea was too self-serving regardless of the benefits to the health delivery process?

Figure 3.5   Chaos: Threat and Opportunity

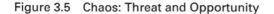

危機

The essential questions for ongoing analysis are: What triggers positive, productive or negative, unproductive behaviors? What positive and negative filters most frequently influence decisions?

PREDICTABLE PHYSICIAN REACTIONS TO CHANGE

The Chinese symbol in Figure 3.5 provides an interesting metaphor for the leader's role in change management. These characters combined mean chaos. The first symbol stands for threat. The second symbol represents opportunity. The two symbols together are the first lesson of the metaphor, that is, all perceived changes cause personal chaos that trigger those behaviors most common to threat.

The major threat to physicians is the loss of control concerning decisions about their practices. Unfortunately, the healthcare economics of the last 20 years has seriously eroded physicians' perception about control of their practices. The degree to which

59

loss of control is perceived determines the amount of reactive aggression.

Physician satisfaction has continued to decline in direct correlation to perceived loss of control. Voluntary attendance at medical staff meetings (about issues other than economics) has declined. Physicians are requesting payment for committee work. These are just some of the behavioral reactions physicians have to perceived threats. A major role of leadership in managing change with physicians is to understand these behaviors as symptoms of the perception of threat to their professional and personal beliefs.

The Chinese symbol in Figure 3.5 helps guide the leader's next decisions. The symbol has two different characters. The second character is "opportunities." The complete metaphor of this symbol is that any crisis is the combination of threat and opportunities. The effective leader of physician change views acting out as a symptom of perceived threat and engages the physicians in a process of discovering the opportunities. Perceived threat creates an environment of negativity and tactical reactions to physician episodes. Engaging physicians in a dialog to discover ways to align their personal and profession goals with corporate strategy moves the dynamic from threat to opportunity.

PHYSICIAN MOTIVATION

Current popular thinking posits that physicians are only interested in money. In fact, physicians (and all other caregivers) are interested in three things: professional respect, control over their work, and money. When respect and control are eliminated from the motivational equation, the default position is money. The reality is that physicians are not only interested in money, but sometimes the only measure of professionalism is money.

The Chinese symbol implies that physicians react to threats with active or passive aggression. We also know that the importance of money is inversely related to being viewed with respect and being allowed to control professional decisions. Managing change with physicians is easier when the set of factors is seen as one phenomenon. The psychodynamics of these factors concern the individual's ego. All humans have an ego and each is unique. However, some consistencies are apparent in the way all egos work. For example, egos will defend themselves against reality that runs counter to history (i.e., filters). Egos need to be fed to maintain strength. If an individual's ego is threatened it will react aggressively. The common term for this reaction is egocentric response. Change management can be viewed as the process of moving the energy of the ego outward. That process has three, stages: *egocentric, rolecentric, and missioncentric.*

Egocentric behavior. Egocentric behavior is characterized by self-interest. Physicians are, many times, criticized for only looking after themselves. When change is misunderstood, unwanted, or out of the control, the first response is "How does this affect me?" This is a predictable response to perceived chaos. Egocentrism will continue until the interest of the person is aligned with the goal of the change process. The best way to deal with egocentrism is to engage the physicians before any change is announced. Anticipation of the egocentric response may not eliminate it entirely but it should lessen its potency.

One engagement technique is to bring together the formal and informal physician leadership and discuss:

1. the proposed change;
2. the reasons for the change; and
3. how the change will affect the physicians' practices.

The role of the leader at this point is to welcome thoughts and feedback. Hopefully, this engagement of the physician leaders takes place early enough in the process to incorporate many of their ideas. Listen to their issues and try to address their self-interests. The more a leader of change can anticipate egocentrism,

61

the easier the leader will be able to move those concerned from egocentrism to rolecentric behavior.

Rolecentric. Rolecentrism is the second stage of reaction to change and concerns job related issues. Common concerns of physicians fixated at the rolecentric level include:

1. Will the location change?
2. How will the changes affect my patients/practice?
3. Who will be responsible if the change interferes with my ability to perform?
4. Will quality be comprised?

When the personal (egocentric) and practice (rolecentric) issues are satisfactorily accommodated, the physicians will enter the missioncentric stage.

Missioncentric behavior. Missioncentrism means that the physicians' personal and professional goals are aligned with the strategic imperatives. Difficulties arise when leadership begins the change process with a discussion about the overall strategy for improving the delivery network and the bottom line. Remember that any change will be perceived by the physician as a threat. This does not mean that the physician is uncooperative or resistant, but that the basic questions about self-interests have not been answered satisfactorily. If the physicians respond with questions about their practice, this indicates they are concerned about their role in the change process.

The lesson for change management is to meet physicians at their level of concern and systematically take them through the first two phases. When you arrive at the third phase (i.e., the shared focus on mission and vision), changes can begin. Attempting to make changes without appreciating the dynamics of these three phases will result in failure, mistrust, and anger.

Figure 3.6   The Easy-to-Hard Change Continuum

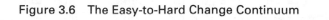
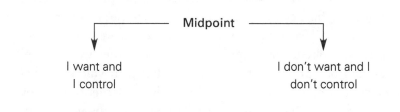

EASY-TO-HARD CHANGE CONTINUUM

Viewing change dynamics on a continuum is one way to under-stand the common negative reactions to change. Change happens all the time. We change easy things such as where we eat lunch or make major life changes such as a new job. Why then is there such a dominant belief that people resist change? The explanation lies in Figure 3.6. People willingly and enthusiasti-cally change those parts of their lives that they want changed and in which they have control over the process. On the other hand, people resist change that they do not want and do not control.

The lessons from this continuum are the essence of managing change with physicians. Change leaders should be sure that any change that involves physicians incorporates their notion of con-trol. If the change triggers a perception that the suits are inter-fering with the physicians' practice, the physicians will fall on the right end of the change management continuum. Also, under-standing the physician groups' filters will eliminate the possibil-ity that they will filter out or discount any aspect that they believe will not improve their practice and filter in or exaggerate those aspects that fit their presuppositions.

A useful preemptive strategy is to engage a small group of phy-sician leaders in a discussion about how to make the vision more relevant to their practice. The guiding principles should be that the vision is non-negotiable and the contribution of the physicians to its success is critical. This focus around the vision blends the needs of the health system and identifies those areas the physicians want and feel they control. Alternative processes that do not engage the physicians in a dialog about what they want or feel they control are doomed to failure. The degree to which the physicians control the movement on those vision elements that they want the most will equal the ease with which the change process will move.

MOTIVATIONAL INFLUENCES ON PERCEPTION AND BEHAVIOR

Behavior is a function of how we view the world. The way individuals view the world is a function of a complex socialization process. The other critical variable that underlies behavior is the arrangement of four motivational influences: recognition, accomplishment, power, and affiliation. The relationship among these four motivational influences determines to a very large degree how we behave.

- Recognition is a need for monetary rewards, promotions, and encouragement. People who have high recognition needs place a high value on respect, bonuses, acclaim, awards, heroes, good pay, and personal goals.
- Accomplishment is the need to find satisfaction in the nature of the work itself. Pride in craftsmanship exists alongside a strong drive for mastery and challenge. An individual with a high accomplishment drive can be characterized as risk taking, results oriented, creative, good with handling pressure, motivated, self-managed, enterprising, and driven.
- Power is the need for competition and a desire for authority and an acceptance of conflict (or, at least, no avoidance of conflict). Words that are often used to describe a power-

influenced individual include: entrepreneurial, good at handling conflict, aggressive, a winner, decisive, high energy, charismatic, challenging, and high maintenance.

• Affiliation focuses on the importance of friendships, loyalty, openness to others, and a readiness to put others ahead of self. Words that describe high-affiliation people are: collective, caring, encouraging, social, safe, trusting, team-focused, fair, and just.

Recognition and affiliation tell us how we relate to work. If recognition motivates us more than accomplishment, we are externally motivated. If accomplishment motivates us more than recognition, we are internally motivated. Knowledge about whether someone is internally or externally motivated is very helpful in designing the appropriate change interaction. For example, externally motivated physicians would want to know the payoff for successful achievement of an objective, whereas an internally motivated individual would want to know whether the objective improves his or her skill mix or where the challenge lies.

The two motivational influences of power and affiliation tell us whether someone prefers to be a team player or is more effective working alone. Also, the relationship between these two factors has a great deal to do with leadership. Behavior that is motivated by power tends to be more aggressive and seem more self-serving. Affiliation-influenced behavior considers loyalty and caring for others as more important than self-interest. Understanding the dynamics of these motivational influences helps the leaders of change explain the reasons for observed behaviors as well as create the best change interventions for the particular motivational pattern.

CONCLUSION

The amount of success with any change management process is a function of perceptual alignment. Everyone involved brings to the process their biases and beliefs about how the world works. These biases and beliefs are a by-product of the individual's socialization process. The sum of all of our experiences produces triggers and filters that determine how we react to any change event.

A trigger is any stimulus or event that elicits a predictable, historically relevant cluster of responses. All behaviors happen because the individuals respond to a situation in ways that worked the past. We learn "correct" responses to a wide variety of events. The behavioral repertoire for a religious service is qualitatively different from the repertoire for an athletic contest. We constantly adjust response patterns to our perception of "correct" behavior. These triggers are learned over time and are very difficult to change. In healthcare organizations, symbols are very important triggers. Logos, titles, and credentials are the most common symbols that control behavior. Understanding organizational symbols is necessary to include in any managed change process in order to determine the strengths of the triggers. Filters are the other powerful dynamic that influences behavior during managed change processes. Filters are those subconscious mechanisms that we use to reinforce our beliefs. Whenever we are confronted with data that contradict our beliefs, we discount that data. And when we observe data that support our position we exaggerate the importance of the data. Humans want to be right. This fact is especially true for highly educated professionals such as physicians.

Change is managed best when the perceptions of all involved are respected as valid. Leaders of change must also realize that regression and egocentrism is a common first reaction to a perceived change. People will embrace change when they understand why it is happening, when they have some control of the change process, and when they see the goal in their best interest.

Chapter Four

CULTURAL FACTORS:
THE EXPERT CULTURE AND
THE COLLECTIVE CULTURE

Great discoveries and achievements invariably involve the cooperation of many minds.

Alexander Graham Bell

He who has a "why" to live for can bear most any "how."

Friedrich Nietzsche

ORPORATE CULTURE IS the personality of the organization. Just as all human beings have personalities, all
organizations have a corporate culture. Whereas personality is the basis for our behavior and decision making, corporate culture is the context for organizational behavior and decision making. Our personalities are the result of a long process
of socialization typically begun by our parents, who had a set of
beliefs or values that they felt were important for us to learn and
use to guide our life's decisions. Our parents systematically taught
us these values through lessons and experience reinforcing those
specific behaviors that were consistent with their values and dis-
ciplining behaviors that were different from their views of good.

67

Essentially, our personality is the sum of experiences that reinforce or weaken behaviors that reflect someone's notion of good
and bad, respectively. The degree to which our behavior is consistent with a set of espoused values equals the strength of our personality. A human being should have only one personality; the
more personalities a person possesses, the more dysfunctional the
individual is in society. The dynamics of personality development
shares many similarities with the creation of a corporate culture.

CORPORATE CULTURE

All organizations have at least one corporate culture—the challenge is to have just one culture, not multiple corporate subcultures. Organizational behavior defines the culture of the organization. In its simplest form, corporate culture is the way things
are done. Healthcare organizations each have a set of espoused
values. The degree to which the behavior displayed on a daily
basis by all, or most, employees demonstrates the strength of the
corporate culture. Therefore more corporate culture is *espoused
values demonstrated by behaviors.* The Walt Disney Company ex-
emplifies a company with a strong corporate culture. Regardless
of whether you visit Disney in Florida or California, the level of
service of the staff is consistent and predictable.

Behavior is driven by a set of values. If the organization's values
are not strong enough to drive individual behavior, the individual's value set is the only basis upon which to define and control
desirable behavior. Values, manifested by behaviors, define the
strength of the culture. However, intangible factors come into
play when creating or strengthening a corporate culture.

TANGIBLE AND INTANGIBLE ELEMENTS

All healthcare factors can be sorted into tangible elements and
the intangible elements. Tangibles are those things that are fairly
easy to measure. Intangibles are those elements that are more

elusive to common measurement but more critical to organizational success. These tangible and intangible factors can be subclassified further into inputs and outputs. For example, on the tangible side, profit is an outcome—you cannot do a "profit." When the business systems are structured so that you spend less than you make, a profit is realized. Another important dynamic among these factors is when the outputs are not at the level you wish (e.g., profit is less than desired), you must go to the inputs that most affect the particular outcome to discover how to alter them to arrive at the desired level. The same fundamental dynamics are imbedded in the intangibles.

Figure 4.1 shows the relationships between and among the main tangible and intangible elements of an organization. Intangibles have both inputs that directly and indirectly affect outputs. Culture is an outcome. You cannot do an outcome—you cannot do corporate culture. The input elements of mission, values, and vision, as processed through leadership, are the most critical. If mission, values, and vision are the ingredients in the recipe for a strong corporate culture, leadership is the quality of the chef who uses the ingredients. Without a great chef the best of ingredients will not come together for a delicious meal. Without the great leadership, the best mission, values, and vision statements cannot come together to produce a strong corporate culture. Leadership is the key and the bridge between leadership and the mission, values, and vision statements is *trust*. Figure 4.2 shows how trust holds the culture together.

TRUST

Trust is the glue that holds organizational culture together. Trust is defined as *the perception of honesty, openness, and reliability/ dependability*. Trust takes a long time to develop and can be broken in a heartbeat. Trust increases as a function of meaningful interactions. The more frequently any group meets over those issues of importance to all, the more trust will be engendered.

Figure 4.1   Relationship Between Tangibles and Intangibles

INPUTS

Tangible	Intangible
Cash	Mission
People	Values
Policy/Procedures	Vision
Strategy	Inspiration
Plant	Leadership Style
Information Systems	Recognition
Communications	Motivation

↓   OUTPUTS   ↓

Tangible	Intangible
Profit	Culture
Market Share	Commitment
Products	Morale
Customer Satisfaction	Job Satisfaction
Growth	Team Spirit
Productivity	Pride/Joy/Trust
Quality	Quality

Leaders involved in managing change with physicians consider trust as so important that they view it as a major strategic imperative. Trusting someone does not mean that you like or care for that individual. There is no correlation between seeing someone as honest, open, and reliable and liking that person. When trust and caring are feelings you have toward an individual, a nice combination results. But liking is not a prerequisite to trust. When dealing with physicians in the change process it is very important that trust be the focus of the interactions. If everyone ends

Figure 4.2   Trust and the Strength of Corporate Culture

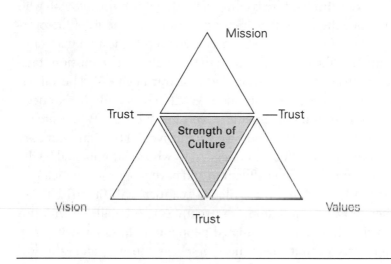

up liking each other, that is wonderful, but not critical to the outcome. Trust is treated differently within collective cultures and expert cultures.

COLLECTIVE CULTURES AND EXPERT CULTURES

The most important factor in understanding how to manage change with physicians and other healthcare providers is the difference between collective cultures and expert cultures. Healthcare systems are comprised of both of these, and many times the difficulty in change management, and even conflicts, can be traced to the fundamental differences between these two cultural phenomena.

COLLECTIVE CULTURES

The collective culture is comprised of highly affiliative staff who embrace the mission, values, and vision statements of the organization. Each of these statements answers a question that is important to those who are collective by nature. The mission statement answers the question, What is our business? The values' statement answers the question, What beliefs underlie our decisions? The vision statement answers the question, Where are we going and how do we know we have arrived? These questions are important to healthcare professionals who are dominated by the motivational profile of affiliation and have progressed in their profession by working in a collegial manner with others. Nurses, therapists, administrators, and many support staff fall into this classification. Highly affiliated people tend to enjoy work environments that put others ahead of self, are trusting, and value loyalty. These professionals like to work in groups, tend to avoid conflict, are not high risk-takers, and tend to be very thin-skinned (i.e., easily injured psychologically). Collective cultures are most discussed in change management literature. However, healthcare has a very important and powerful group that does not conform to the definition of collectives. This group behaves like experts and prefers the expert culture environment. This group is physicians.

EXPERT CULTURES

Expert cultures possess very different characteristics and dynamics from collective cultures. Expert cultures do not need mission statements or value statements. Trust may or may not exist—indeed it usually does not exist outside a very narrow range of clear expectations for performance. Expert cultures are found in engineering firms, architectural firms, multispecialty law firms, and the profession of medicine. Expert cultures are characterized by individualized behavior that is motivated primarily by self-interest.

Unlike collective cultures, wherein affiliation is the major motivational influence, expert cultures are dominated by the motivational influences of accomplishment and power. The reasons people are attracted to collective or expert cultures are found in their respective socialization experiences. Physicians are experts, whereas, for the most part, other clinicians are collectives. Their chosen professions require very different work-life experiences.

Characteristics of an expert culture individual. Starting at a very early age, children who wish to become doctors compete for grades. Grade school and high school become opportunities to demonstrate academic and leadership potential. Selection to a prestigious college becomes an obsession. The choice of medical schools in turn will determine to a large degree the resident match. After completing residency and the medical boards, the decisions of where to practice and in what specialty has a lot to do with professional and financial success. There is no place or time in this more than 20-year process where success resulted from teamwork. At each point, success was determined by outperforming the competition. Achievement, risk-taking, stamina, intense focus, quick decision making, and personal accountability were some of the main characteristics that were consistently reinforced. Consensus building, interdependency, following orders, and sacrificing self-interest for the greater good are not often found in the socialization process of experts. A simple metaphor shows the difference between the expert culture and the collective culture.

A mythical description of physician team building potential is "herding cats." A better description of an effective physician team is a golf team. The only way for the United States to win the Ryder Cup is for each member of the team to perform at his personal best. Compare this to winning the NBA championship. The Los Angeles Lakers were comprised of outstanding basketball players for many years before Phil Jackson took over as coach. However, until they learned to suppress their expert needs for interdependency, they did not perform at their highest potential. Healthcare delivery is comprised of both experts and collectives. The challenge of leadership is to create an environment in which both cultures can manifest their needs for the greater good—serving the healthcare needs of the community. This means that change management strategies for collectives must include group work that is contextualized in mission, values, and vision. The change management strategies for experts (i.e., physicians) need to focus on a shared vision wherein the physician can see his or her self-interest manifest in the successful achievement of the vision. Self-interest versus group interest delineates the expert culture from the collective culture. An unusual example may be instructive—The Dennis Rodman Syndrome.

The Dennis Rodman syndrome. Former professional basketball player Dennis Rodman is an extreme example of how the expert's need to feed self-interest is his or her main motivation. Any other motivational interventions that do not incorporate personal (or in Rodman's case narcissistic) needs will fail. Dennis is an expert at one thing—collecting basketballs off the backboard.

When Dennis played with the San Antonio Spurs, the coach attempted to motivate him by trying to have him behave using the values of David Robinson. David Robinson is a wonderful human being—very caring and giving. Trying to make Dennis use the same values as David was doomed from the start. When Dennis moved to the Chicago Bulls, a very different approach was used by coach Phil Jackson. Coach Jackson understood that the only way to motivate an expert is to engage his or her self-interest. He told Dennis that if he collected basketballs off the rim and gave them to his teammate Michael Jordan, he would be paid an obscene amount of money. Phil Jackson never incorporated values into Dennis' motivational formula. The formula to motivate Dennis is the only one that works with experts: identify a common, shared vision in which the expert sees his or her self-interests being met when the vision is achieved.

Figure 4.3   Comparison of Collective and Expert Cultures

Collective—High Affiliative	Expert—High Power
Thin skinned	Thick skinned
Very sensitive to injury	High risk
Injure: commission or omission	Must win or L-L
Long memory for injury	Insensitive to collectives
Risk averse	Results versus process
Process versus outcome	Fast "clear" decisions
Change causes "FUD"	Self-interest first
High need for recognition	Like to lead
Conflict resolution motif	Conflict motif
• Denial	• Direct confrontation
• Passive aggression	
• Explosion	
Malignant = Cynic/Victim	Malignant = Narcissism

NEITHER CULTURE IS RIGHT OR WRONG

Figure 4.3 outlines the differences between collective and expert cultures. An important point vis-à-vis collective and expert cultures is that there is no right or wrong with either of these motifs. A common reflex is to denigrate the experts' desire to see their self-interest in the shared purpose and support those who work in groups with shared values. They are both unique to the socialization of the expert or the collective. These behaviors are "hard-wired" into the person. Wishing they were different is useless. Change leaders understand, and respect, the unique dynamics of both cultures and use the interactions that most fit the needs of the expert and the collective. Corporate culture is the context in which any change is perceived as good or bad. This

75

Figure 4.4   Culture Characteristics

	Aligned	Misaligned
Collective	Values-Based Behaviors	Fear
	Openness	Uncertain
	Innovation	Doubt
	Joy and/or Pride	Small Sub-Culture
	Customer Satisfaction	Minimum Behavior
Expert	Vision-Based Focus	Egocentric
	Collegiality	Economic Focus
	Feel Respected	Personal Autonomy
	Feel in Control	Conflict
	Collaboration	Anger

perception is a function of whether the individuals' motivation is influenced more by affiliation (collective culture) or accomplishment and power (expert culture). The main goal of leadership is to align the collectives and the experts. Figure 4.4 describes the reactions of aligned and misaligned culture.

CULTURAL FACTORS AND MERGERS

Problems often arise when trying to merge healthcare corporations that have different cultures. Too often merger decisions are based only on tangible elements such as increased market share, economies of scale, and decreased competition. However, while most mergers are executed on the basis of the tangibles, most failed mergers are the result of the intangibles—most often a clash of corporate cultures. Merging cultures is difficult when collective behaviors are the only behaviors considered. Mergers that include medical staffs and medical groups present a complex dimension to the process.

Collective cultures must create new mission, value, and vision statements. The merging entities must design ways to communicate these new statements in ways that increases trust. An unpleasant history of failed healthcare mergers just in the last decade has emerged. Each of these failures can be traced to conflicts in one or more intangibles. A significant number of mergers have had some success in merging the collective cultures but have yet to make any, or just minimal, progress with the expert physician culture. Following are some models and examples that may help explain why mergers succeed or fail, as well as some models that address the differences between collective and expert cultures.

MERGER MODELS: COLLECTIVE AND EXPERT CULTURES

THE EQUAL BLEND MODEL

Figure 4.5 shows the scheme that most merger plans use. Two relatively equal hospitals (many times a Catholic one and a community one) create a new, coequal entity. The new entity is very often given some new name that makes sense only to the people who created it (e.g., Intergalactic Health System). The underlying myth of this approach is that everything should be equal and the physicians and the community will understand clearly the new mission, value, and vision statements. The structure of the equal blend model requires that half of the board members be taken from one entity and half from the other. The executive team and middle managers are selected using the same "Solomonesque" technique of half-and-half. The parity mentality, while very easy to design and consistent with good democratic values, seldom works. Rather than creating an efficient new healthcare delivery entity, gridlock results. Highly affiliative

Figure 4.5   Equal Blend Model

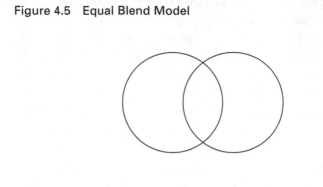

persons are attracted to this model because it seems so fair. Problems begin to emerge when difficult decisions need to be made about service realignment, staff adjustments, and new business development. Pleasantries turn to frustration at the decision-making point because the leaders are so embedded in their initial hospital loyalty. Physicians during this process are usually very verbal about how bad the merger idea was in the first place, negating any hope of engaging them in building a new future.

THE BIG DOG–LITTLE DOG MODEL

The merger model in Figure 4.6 is really a take-over model. No matter what euphemisms are used to create the notion of a partnership, the fact remains that the larger or smaller in size but more aggressive organization will determine the culture. This can be an efficient method for creating the desirable culture. That is, the merger tells the mergee the decision rules. If the mergee does not agree, it is replaced. This model is more common in non-healthcare industries, for example, banking and manufacturing. The model, although efficient, poses many dangerous problems,

Figure 4.6   Big Dog–Little Dog Model

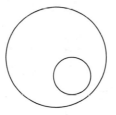

especially for healthcare. The model requires an autocratic, non-engaging approach.

Autocratic approaches have some predictable dynamics. Their biggest problem is that they reinforce the autocratic. The people in charge actually think they have done something and have done it fast. The fact is there may be some immediate, observable changes in the tangibles elements of structure, such as the number of full-time employees, the amount of pay, etc. However, while the autocrat is pointing to these changes with pride, a furtive and powerful dynamic is at work—passive aggression. Autocratic change methodologies always produce passive aggressive behavior and passive aggression will *always* destroy the merger in the long run. It is the silent killer.

This model is especially ineffective with buying or merging physician practices. Physicians are motivated to a large degree by accomplishment and power. Autocratic techniques to control physician behavior never have and never will work. A great enthusiasm for buying practices existed for a period of time. There were (and still are) seminars on controlling physician practice behavior. The autocratic attempts at merging expert cultures have

79

Figure 4.7   Satellite Model

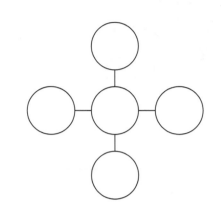

proved to be a fool's journey. You do not control experts—you engage them in a process of mutual self-interest.

THE SATELLITE MODEL

The model in Figure 4.7 works for both collective and expert cultures. Mergers are designed to improve economics through the benefits of size. Most mergers are designed to create a new or strengthen a current economic engine. Multicorporate health-care delivery systems seldom seek to create a single corporate culture across all entities and sites. However, this runs counter to the common thinking: we are one organization, therefore we need one set of mission, values, and vision statements.

Newly merged entities are designed to improve the financial and business aspects of care delivery. These corporate entities do not see patients, and rarely find a physician or nurse at the corporate office. Corporate offices should not try to create a single

Figure 4.8   Chaos Model

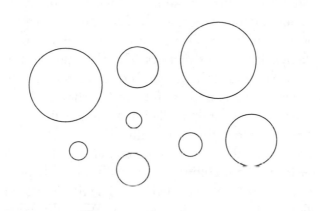

culture; they should use some of their resources to increase the strength of the local cultures currently in place.

Variations on this model can be incorporated into planning depending on the special factors of a specific system. The most common variation is to have a common mission and values statement across the system but allow each entity to create its own vision statement or at least its own strategic plan. This promotes corporate consistency and permits the unique aspects of the various sites to be expressed in strategy. This model incorporates the accomplishment and power needs of the experts as well as the group needs of the collectives.

THE CHAOS MODEL

Chaos is the most common response to mergers (see Figure 4.8). The staff at the merging entities have little trust in the new corporation. The enthusiasm displayed by the senior executives for the new corporation is met with fear and distrust by those who do not know if they will fit into the future of the new entity. They default to what they are sure of—their personal value systems. Chapter 3 discussed the notions of egocentric and rolecentric responses to unknown change processes. The chaos model predictably elicits these dynamics. The challenge for leadership is to anticipate these behaviors and create a communication system that helps the staff understand how they fit into the new entity. However, the major difficulty is that the merging entities divide themselves into multiple subcultures.

Sometimes it is useful to remember that the whole body of knowledge about cultures began with the study of tribes. The chaos model of organizational behavior reflects some of the basic understandings about tribal behavior. When threatened, people tend to cluster around those with similar values and concerns. During the chaos stage of organizational transformation, tribes emerge. Tribes may include nurse tribes, doctor tribes, administration tribes, and so on. These tribes become the base for individual decision making. The thinking goes something like this: I have no idea what *they* are up to therefore; I will stay with those I trust and wait to see what happens. Tribal behavior is very common during a massive change like a merger. It is the behavioral reflex to perceived chaos. Although it is predictable, effective leaders try to move from the perception of chaos to commitment to the new entity, from tribes to a focused work force, as soon as possible. The longer the tribes are allowed to exist, the more difficult they are to change.

THE EXPERT MODEL

The expert model of cultural formation is best illustrated by a series of circles lined up in orderly rows (see Figure 4.9). The lesson of this model is that the integrity of the individual is protected along side coequals, all of whom wish to achieve a predetermined goal.

Figure 4.9 Expert Model

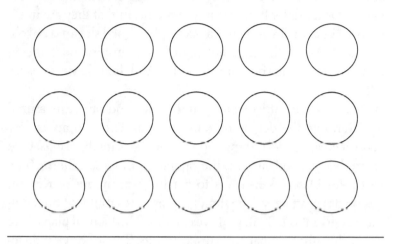

The key to making this model work is the time spent engaging the experts in the creation of a goal that they all see as important to their personal interests. The issues of shared mission and core values are not the factors that make this model work. In fact, emphasis on mission and values will contaminate this model to the point that it may not work at all. The only cultural element that makes the expert model work is shared vision. The dynamic which makes the expert model work is allowing the expert to control the process as it relates to his or her practice and respecting his or her judgment in terms of ongoing decision making. Experts respond well to change processes when they feel in control of the decisions that most affect them and feel professional respect throughout the development and implementation of the process.

THE POWER OF VISION

All visions have three characteristics. They are inspirational, they are directional, and they are manageable. The more effective vision statements tend to be short. However, some people, in an attempt to be efficient, convert their vision statements into slogans. Slogans differ from vision statements in that they are inspirational but not directional. For example, a good slogan is Nike's: Just Do It! While this statement can be very inspirational, the direction is anything you want "it" to be. And, how do we measure "doing it?"

Visions inspire, drive strategy and tactics, and can be measured to determine the degree of achievement. The military is very good at creating clear, inspirational, and measurable visions. One example of a good vision is the operation in Desert Storm. The vision for Desert Storm was to get Iraq's army out of Kuwait. Vision drives strategy. The strategic plan was a multinational military intervention. Strategy drives tactics. The tactical plans were defined by the combat and support units. Tactics drive individual performance. The plans were so precise that each military person knew exactly what had to be done to achieve the goals of the plan. Vision to strategy to tactics to individual performance is the power of visions. They convert overall corporate expectations to precise individual behaviors. The people who must make the vision real understand their contribution to overall success. Their behavior is contextualized in a greater good rather than personal self-interest or survival.

Organizations without a vision. Organizations that do not use vision as the context for change default to retrovisioning (i.e., tactical reactions and survival behaviors) and tactical responses. This behavioral pattern is more reflected in the military action in Vietnam. The espoused vision of the war in Vietnam was to *Stop Communism.* While this statement may have had an inspirational effect on some in Washington D.C., there was no direction.

The vision was too vague to drive a comprehensive strategic plan and the tactical plans seem to be reactive. The result of these factors was to create a combat force that had no greater good to inspire them and, therefore, defaulted to survival. This same dynamic happens far too often in healthcare organizations. The vision either does not exist or is too vague to inspire individual behavior toward a greater good. The staff default to retrovisioning. They do not know how they fit into the future, so they reproduce past behavior and hope that they keep their jobs. This predictable reaction to an uninspiring workplace is very toxic. Staff members are tired, stressed, and frightened. These are good people who want to do the right thing but are in an environment that forces them to be egocentric.

The Desert Storm and Vietnam examples convey many lessons for physician partnerships. Desert Storm was the coming together of many countries with very diverse cultures, many of whom could not speak each others' language. Some of these countries were historic enemies. All the separate, diverse, country-specific issues were subordinated to the greater good as perceived in a common, shared vision. Unlike Vietnam where, even though the forces were mainly from the United States, and therefore spoke the same language as well as having a shared history, the lack of a shared vision forced the military personnel into holding actions. Whether behavior is egocentric, survival focused, decentered, or outwardly focused is a function of the degree to which people see their contribution to the greater good. This greater good possesses obvious benefits to all involved. Self-interest and corporate interest are aligned and obvious. Keep in mind that "liking each other" and even "trust" are not necessary when bringing experts together to achieve a shared vision.

Long-term behaviors. The final lesson from Desert Storm that is consistent with expert cultures relates to long-term behaviors. When the vision of removing the Iraqi army from Kuwait was achieved, those involved returned to their homelands. The biases and prejudices that existed before the war were back in place. Little if any positive carry-over ocurred. The same is true with expert culture dynamics. Just because a group of physicians came together for a particular strategic thrust in which they saw their needs being met does not, in any way, suggest that the next effort will be supported. The difference between collective and expert cultures is that collective cultures have a common mission, values, and vision and build trust on the basis of successful results. Expert cultures are successful only in connection with a specific vision wherein self-interest is obvious. Each time you wish to engage a group of physicians (or other experts), it's like starting over. You cannot generalize from one successful venture to the next. The dynamics of collaboration more suit experts in a change process than the transformational efforts that are effective with collectives.

CONCLUSION

The definition of collaboration is a mutually beneficial relationship with clear roles that is entered into by two or more individuals and/or corporations to achieve common goals. Collaborative efforts are successful when there is a clear understanding of relationships and goals; a jointly developed structure and shared responsibilities; authority and accountabilities are accepted; and, a mutually developed vision in which each member sees his or her self-interest.

To attempt collective culture change techniques with experts is frustrating and, in fact, counterproductive. The main difference between expert techniques and collective techniques is the respective roles of vision and values. Experts will support any change effort wherein the goal or vision includes their self-interest. Collectives, on the other hand, are more concerned about shared values. Collectives, like experts, want to see how they fit into the future, but more importantly, collectives want to align with a group with similar beliefs. Experts do not make shared values a prerequisite for commitment. When experts share the corporate values, the change process has less tension but shared values alone will not mobilize experts. Successful leaders focus on a shared vision for both experts and collectives and spend time on shared values for collectives.

Chapter Five

HEALTHCARE IN A
CHANGING WORLD

A learning organization is a place where people are continually discovering how they create their reality, and how they
can change it.

Peter Senge

T HE PACE OF change is progressing exponentially.
Marked instability in the environment follows accelerating developments in transportation, communication,
and information. These infrastructure technologies govern the
flow of goods, people, money, and information. The road to success demands adaptability and flexibility. As reviewed in chapter
1, consumerism, competition, and technological innovation are
driving change. Innovation and creativity have become more
important than perfectibility. To be economically sustainable,
healthcare providers have to forge intimate relationships with
their customers and be able to "create on the fly."

Cause-and-effect linkages exist among beliefs about how the
world works, how society is structured, the economic system that

supports those social structures, and the organizational structures and styles of management that support the economic system. During the middle ages, world views were tied to religious beliefs. The clergy provided in magical and religious frameworks an interpretation of how the world worked. Subsequently, the renaissance and the scientific revolution occurred and Newtonian physics became the basis for interpreting the laws of the universe.

THE PATH TO CHANGE

In a Newtonian world, discovering universal laws allows for predictability and control of the environment. Breaking things down into progressively smaller parts and understanding each of these smaller parts allows an understanding of the whole. The universe is seen as a machine and the whole is the sum of its component parts.

Today, quantum physics is displacing Newtonian physics as a way of understanding how the universe works. Unlike a Newtonian world of universal laws, a quantum world sees things as changeable and dependent on context and relationships. Whether subatomic elements behave as particles or waves depends on how they are measured. Properties are emergent and observer-dependent and the whole is not the sum of its parts. The linear world of cause and effect gives way to a world that is now seen as nonlinear, nonlocal, and self organizing (Wheatley 1994).

As these world views have changed, so have the structures of contemporaneous economic organizations. From a social and economic perspective, western societies have passed through a number of progressive societal revolutions, from hunters and gatherers to an agrarian and artisan society, through the industrial revolution, the information revolution, and now the bioterial revolution. (The last of these relates to the emerging ability to not just adapt ourselves to our existing environment, but to be able to genetically transform who we are and to create *de novo* new elements designed to meet specific needs.) Each of these revolutions is related to changing views about how the universe works.

During the preindustrial, agrarian period, artisans comprised cottage industries. With the advent of the scientific method, a Newtonian perspective led to the organizational and management styles of the industrial revolution.

Currently, industrial models are failing to provide the flexibility and adaptability necessary to successfully respond to the rapidly changing environmental demands of the information revolution. As Newtonian physics gives way to quantum physics, new organizational models better suited to the needs of the information age are beginning to emerge. Managing context and relationships is replacing hierarchical command and control.

Even as the healthcare industry is moving from an artisan-based cottage industry through managed care's attempts to impose industrial process controls (the industrial revolution), a new design is needed that emphasizes diversification, decentralization, segmentation of the market place, and other adaptations that reflect the transition of control from the providers of healthcare services to healthcare consumers (information revolution). With this transition, new styles of leadership and management are needed in the pursuit of enhancing the adaptability and sustainability of healthcare organizations. We will describe how the stakeholders in the healthcare industry form a complex adaptive system and why, given the exponential pace of change, the future is not only unpredictable, but also unknowable. Several ways in which leadership and management are changing in response to pressures to adapt to this rapidly changing environment will be examined.

FROM COTTAGE INDUSTRY TO INDUSTRIAL MODEL

Hospital-based services have evolved through several economic models. They began as charity-supported, often religious-based organizations. Healthcare services were limited to comforting the sick, and hospitals were places where those who could not afford to remain at home went to die. With the advent of anesthesia, surgical interventions became possible, and hospitals became places where persons could be restored to health. At that time hospital services became truly fee-for-service; patients were expected to pay what they could afford for the services provided. With the advent of employment-based health insurance, hospitals began to do business in a cost plus manner that continued until the advent of Medicare's prepayment system. Now the amount of those prepayments have reduced and are fixed in advance, and efficiency of operations has become critical for creating positive operating margins.

Because economic access to healthcare in the United States is significantly employment based, as economic competition became globalized, the perception that healthcare resources are unlimited came to an end. Businesses in the United States found it progressively more difficult to successfully compete globally because of the amount of overhead expenses they allocate to providing healthcare benefits to their employees. In an attempt to control healthcare costs, managed care was born. The initial response has been the equivalent of a belated industrial revolution in healthcare. Attempts have been made to aggregate hospitals to achieve economies of scale and to apply industrial process control methods to healthcare through the use of pathways and guidelines, utilization review, and case management initiatives. Techniques intended to reduce variation in healthcare are analogous to those applied to the mass production of automobiles. When artisans make cars, parts are not interchangeable. With mass production, parts are interchangeable, results predictable, and efficiencies and effectiveness of products controllable.

The industrial model in healthcare. Today's healthcare organizations are structured according to an industrial model of management and control. Span of control is critical. The CEO sits at the top of a branching hierarchy of management that progressively communicates the strategic and tactical decisions to the workforce. Most industrial-age organizations adopted this assembly line approach to management. Frederick Taylor, an engineer, viewed workers and their tasks as cogs in a machine. The tasks were specifically designed and the employees were controlled by management who were charged with progressively assembling the whole. The production process was broken down into discreet parts or functions and workers were instructed on how to efficiently perform their isolated function. Parts and workers were interchangeable and needed management to achieve predictable results (Zimmerman 1998).

This organizational model works well in stable and predictable environments where replication of predictable outcomes determine economic success. Paradigms are stable, and the road to continuing success equates to doing what has made you successful in the past. It is an effective organizational model when information is difficult to assemble and can only be collated by the few individuals at the top of the organizational hierarchy. Information is a source of power, and only those at the top have the complete picture and, therefore, the ability to make strategic and tactical decisions on behalf of the organization. Only the necessary information is moved down into the organization through management. In a similar fashion, accountability moves up the organizational hierarchy. Each successive layer of management evaluates the layer below.

NEW MODELS FOR A CHANGING ENVIRONMENT

The ability to almost instantaneously access information has accelerated the pace of change and destabilized the environment. Now the road to success demands adaptability and flexibility. Consumerism is fueled in part by the ease of access to information.

93

To be successful, persons who work with consumers must have access to real-time measurement feedback and customer needs must be anticipated. Successful companies provide this information to the workforce and allow them to make decisions. Diversification, decentralization, and access to information are characteristics of organizations that succeed in rapidly changing environments. When these capabilities are present, the need for span of control is markedly reduced as information is rapidly and widely shared and accountability becomes clear as everyone throughout the organization can view how everyone else is performing. These same transforming forces are impacting healthcare. As in other industries, in order to successfully adapt, healthcare organizations must relinquish their hierarchical, command and control structures.

Physicians as artisans. Despite these transformational changes, physicians continue to function as artisans in a guild. For physicians, the cottage industry of medicine is only now beginning to change. In the physician's world, even when they practice in large groups, healthcare is practiced one patient–one physician at a time. The service is believed to be as unique as the products of any preindustrialized artisan. Managed care (translated as managed cost) has sought to override this behavior and reduce variation through the standardization of healthcare processes and to control healthcare costs through application of an industrial model.

Healthcare and the industrial revolution. People are not cars, and biological systems do not perform as mechanical systems. The emergence of the information revolution has condensed the time period of healthcare's passage through the industrial revolution. When the consumer's access to information is similar to that of the producer of the goods or services, the power differential between them disappears. Economic competition increases and informed consumers begin to make choices based on their needs and expectations. Producers are now forced to customize their offerings, segment their markets, and create distinctions that are valued by those market segments. It no longer remains a cost plus world, but rather an economy in which value is determined by worth to the consumer, not by cost of production. Patient and physician rejection of the managed cost characteristics of managed care are reflected in the emerging emphasis on mass customization and perceived individualization of healthcare services. The growth in point-of-service plans also reflects this trend. Healthcare is passing through the industrial revolution and the information revolution at "warp speed," as its organizational models begin to reflect changes in other industries.

INTERDEPENDENCIES IN HEALTHCARE

Individual stakeholders and stakeholder groups do not exist in isolation from others in their industry. The definition of complex adaptive systems and several examples of interdependency will demonstrate these linkages and their consequences. In this context suboptimization of the whole is an important principle to understand. Interpreting the world through the perspective of quantum physics offers an opportunity to better understand how the applications of these principles to organizational design and management allows organizations to become more adaptable and improve the chances of sustaining their organizational purpose.

COMPLEX ADAPTIVE SYSTEMS[1]

Healthcare is part of a complex adaptive system (Zimmerman and Plsek 1998). It is complex because many separate agencies or subsystems make up the entire system of healthcare. There are physicians and hospitals, nurses and other professional and ancillary personnel, alternative providers, insurance companies, employers, legislatures, lawyers, pharmaceutical firms, technology development companies, and educational institutions, just to name a few.

It is adaptive because each of the separate agencies act to maximize its own position by responding to changes in its immediate environment according to its own decision-making rules. The consequences of those decisions have variable and unpredictable consequences for the other agencies. The output of any one agency, in a nonlinear fashion, becomes input for other. In a linear system, A affects B, which affects C. In a nonlinear system, A affects B, which in turn can affect A and D and any other component in an unpredictable manner. An example of this dynamic is the unforeseen consequences of the Balanced Budget Act on many healthcare agencies. The federal legislature acted in response to its perceived need to balance the budget, rein in the rising costs of healthcare for Medicare beneficiaries, and curb some of the abuses it saw in the home health and nursing home industries. Consequent to this legislation the five-year plans that called for investing in the continuum of care by building an infrastructure of home health care services and transitional care nursing beds unraveled. Who could have predicted that turn of events?

Healthcare as an ecosystem. Complex adaptive systems behave more like ecosystems than machines. Interdependencies, both identified and unforeseen exist. Each agency acts independently in response to changes in its immediate environment. Those adaptations effect it and other agencies within that environment causing further change in the environment and causing others to react. A constant dialectic of change and a progressive evolution of environmental complexity evokes from its component subsystems a progressively more complex state of adaptation. The results are unpredictable and unknowable and makes the very notion of a five-year plan ridiculous.

The tragedy of the commons.[2] The allegory of the tragedy of the commons illustrates the interdependencies of individuals who are part of the same system (Senge 1990). In this allegory, a community sustains itself by raising sheep. Each family raises its own flock, but the only place where all the sheep can graze is an area shared by all the families called the commons. Who suffers if one of the shepherds allows his flock to overgraze the commons? By analogy, when a single constituent in the larger healthcare system makes a decision that is designed to selfishly enhance its own position, everyone, including that constituent, ultimately suffers. It is an ecosystem, and the entire system will act to try to reestablish balance. Eliminating or disadvantaging a component of that ecosystem can have many unforeseen effects. The expedient decisions made today to enhance the short-term needs of one member can ultimately serve to harm not just the larger system but also that very decision maker. This phenomenon occurs repeatedly when governments make policy in response to a perceived immediate need, only to find that the policy ultimately creates tomorrow's crisis. Other examples of how interdependencies link members of complex adaptive systems are seen in the consequences of destroying coral reefs or of polluting the environment.

Suboptimization of the whole. For an entire system to operate at maximum efficiency, no component of that system can operate at maximum efficiency. This principle was discussed in Chapter 2 and is equally applicable to a discussion of the interdependency of subsystems within the ecology of an encompassing larger system. When healthcare organizations apply productivity indices to the evaluation and reward systems of their individual departments, they invariably suboptimize the integrated performance of the whole. The individual department managers seek to optimize their performance and put into place operations designed to buffer their department against risks that their performance optimums will be compromised by potential deficiencies created by

97

others over whom they have no direct control. This invariably adds complexity and variability to those processes that span departments. The more important measure of performance should be one that assesses the integrated performance of various constituents in accomplishing the final shared output. This would promote teamwork and help integrate and orchestrate the various processes that contribute to the final end product.

Complex adaptive systems and quantum physics.[3] Complexity science, sometimes referred to as "new science," is rooted in quantum physics. It is a world where relationships and context determine properties. Unlike the reductionistic world of Newtonian physics where an understanding of the parts predicts the properties of the whole; in the quantum world, reassembling parts leads to a whole with emergent properties that are not knowable in advance. For example, there is no way that a thorough understanding of the gases hydrogen and oxygen can predict the properties of water, or understanding the behavioral characteristics of a single ant can predict the complex interactive behaviors that emerge within an ant colony. In complex adaptive systems, adaptations emerge in response to changing environmental demands. Because the nature of these emergent adaptations is unpredictable, the role of leadership evolves into managing the relationships and context out of which these changes emerge. Gareth Morgan has popularized the metaphorical analogy: "Farmers don't grow crops, they create conditions in which crops grow" (Zimmerman and Plsek 1998).

CHANGING STYLES OF LEADERSHIP

New forms of organizational design and new styles of leadership have emerged in response to the growing complexity of a rapidly changing external environment. Complexity science supported by the changing perspectives that have evolved from a world view transformed by quantum physics has become a new metaphor for understanding how to successfully adapt to the demands of a progressively more complex environment. Some new concepts have emerged, including:

- understanding self-organization and emergence;
- resolving paradox;
- applying action-based research;
- promoting a learning organization;
- the special nature of professional bureaucracies;
- the nature of group resistance to change; and
- the use of metaphors to transform organizations.

SELF-ORGANIZATION AND EMERGENCE[4]

Margaret Wheatley writes of the applications of complexity science to organizational leadership and management and uses the aftermath of the bombing of the federal building in Oklahoma City as an example of two characteristics of complex adaptive systems—self-organization and emergence (Wheatley 1994). Almost immediately after the bombing the entire world could watch what happened on television through the eyes of CNN. What they saw was a remarkable and well-coordinated effort at finding, stabilizing, transporting, and treating the injured. The immediate and coordinated response impressed persons in other cities who were charged with the responsibility for emergency preparedness. Many contacted the Oklahoma City government to obtain a copy of their disaster plan however, there was no disaster plan. In fact, what happened in response to this tragedy was self-organizing and emergent. Wheatley observes that when individuals who share a common purpose are given access to all the necessary information and are allowed to engage in "soulful dialog," self-organization occurs. Unpredictable solutions emerge. This style of leadership is better suited to rapidly changing environments and far more successful than command and control approaches (Pfeffer 1998; Belasco and Stayer 1993).[5,6]

99

RESOLVING PARADOX[7]

Gareth Morgan suggests that successful leadership involves appreciating the value of surfacing and managing paradox (Morgan 1997). New ideas challenge the status quo and are resisted by those who benefit from the current system. Each paradigm has merit in its own right. This conflict creates the "yeah ... buts" that surface in debates over the value of new approaches. Persons listening to the new proposal respond to the perceived advantages with a sequence of acknowledged "yeahs," but then quickly follow with the "buts" that reflect the advantages of the current way of behaving. Focusing on how to resolve the "yeah ... buts" allows the discovery of new ways of advancing change. What resolution can be proposed that will incorporate advantages of the old with incremental advantages of the new? Resolving this paradox is one way that creative change can occur.

Morgan advises that we focus on those areas in which we have the potential to assert influence. He postulates that about 15 percent of your total range of activities involves circumstances in which you have the capacity to be influential. It is in these areas that you should seek to focus your efforts. Change within complex adaptive systems is nonlinear. The magnitude of the output is disproportional to the input. Because of the nonlinearity of change, small changes in these areas can have a disproportionately large impact on the entire organization.

Changes within your sphere of influence can be further enhanced if they are directed at points of high leverage. Make a list of negatives that exist within your sphere of influence, answer the question, "why does this occur," and draw arrows to other items on the list that are causal. You will almost always find that two or three primary causes emerge. The other items on the list are only symptomatic manifestations of these more primary root causes. If you can focus your change efforts within these few points of highest leverage, you can maximize the impact of the proposed changes. In addition successes within your sphere of influence may sometimes serve as prototypes of change for others. In this way, you can also realize a disproportionate impact on the entire organization.

ACTION-BASED RESEARCH[8]

Action-based research is a key to creating change. Also termed rapid cycle improvement, this methodology, promoted by the Institute for Healthcare Improvement, is a useful model for piloting new ideas that can potentially transform how work is done. In the rapid cycle improvement approach, you first identify and continually assess the following two measurements:

- a global measure that assesses the integrated larger goal to be achieved, and
- a measure of a component process that you want to improve that is very short term, easy to collect, and that assesses the results of your focused intervention.

An improvement initiative is acted upon and the short-term impact of that change is continually assessed in a way to guide further refinements. In this way you act, measure the impact, interpret the results, and continue to move forward, creating "on the fly." It is an action-oriented approach to making and assessing change. The more global measure is essential to ensure that any component change does not result in a suboptimization of the more encompassing objective.

THE LEARNING ORGANIZATION[9]

Because the world is transforming so rapidly it is impossible for organizational leaders to make predictions with certainty. The amount of available information and the complexities of environmental interactions and interdependencies exceed the capacity of the human mind to manage all of the variables. How can you position your organization for success? How do you nurture an environment that is adaptable and flexible? One answer is to cultivate a learning organization.

Adaptable organizations that are capable of changing and successfully evolving, as described by Peter Senge (1998), are like gardens. They are not organizations that are tightly directed the top down. Those organizations are all about control. They are seen as machines that operators can control in the service of its owner's objectives. When change is necessary, the boss hires a mechanic who can bring in new parts and fix it.

Senge suggests that rather than needing mechanics, you need gardeners; rather than trying to drive change, you cultivate change. A willingness to change and a sense of openness, reciprocity, and even vulnerability are required. Deep change comes only through real personal growth, through learning and unlearning. Relationships, teamwork, and trust are essential to effective operations (Senge 1998). In top down imposed change the best you can hope for is compliance. Deep change only comes about when people act out of commitment. Commitment comes about when people determine that you are asking them to do something that they really care about. Senge states that people want to have fun being part of a team that does meaningful things that make them proud.

PROFESSIONAL BUREAUCRACIES

Hospital organizations are professional bureaucracies and differ significantly from nonprofessional bureaucracies. For example, physicians, who allocate variable expenses, usually are not employed by the organization and are not under its direct control. Physicians are not often directly affected by the organization's economic success or failure. Clinicians and healthcare organizations distrust each other because they operate from different assumptions. Nurses, who are employed by the organization, have dual loyalties. They must comply with the wishes of their employer and adhere to the ethics of their profession. Professional standards and ethics influence individual behavior and therefore significantly affect organizational behaviors.

Physicians and personal failure. Failure is not accepted in the healthcare profession and is perceived as individual incompetence. By expecting perfection from themselves, healthcare professionals create an environment that refuses to openly challenge current behaviors because any possible deficiencies could be interpreted as personal inadequacy. Chris Argyris observes that people who rarely experience failure do not know how to deal with it. This reinforces the normal human tendency to reason defensively (Argyris 1991). Professionals are especially threatened by the prospect of critically examining their own role in the organization. They insist that fault lies with others and cannot see their contribution to the problem. Professionals want to remain in control, maximize winning and minimize losing, suppress negative feelings, and be as rational as possible. "The purpose is to avoid embarrassment or threat, feeling vulnerable or incompetent" (Argyris 1991). This behavior is a perfect description of how physicians interact with others in the healthcare setting and often characterizes the discussions between physicians and senior hospital personnel. Physicians are predisposed to work out their problems in isolation, display their best face in public, overemphasize short-term results, and infrequently admit they do not know something. This quick-fix mentality makes them system-blind and explains why today's problems come from yesterday's solutions.

Change requires letting go. Individuals have to be able to let go of current beliefs and attitudes in order to change. They must learn to become vulnerable, and be willing to examine their operating assumptions, and to own their contribution to the present circumstances. Dialog should be valued by balancing advocacy and inquiry as a method for learning. Do they truly understand the other person's position, or only their view of the other's position? Are they willing to reveal the reasoning behind their position and to invite criticism of its logic? This is very difficult for physicians who are frequently placed in positions of authority. In making critical decisions on behalf of their patients they must be secure in their beliefs. Therefore, they are predisposed to behave paternalistically and are strongly opinionated.

Patients desperately need to believe their physician, and the physician needs to believe that his or her position is correct. How could they look at themselves if they felt that they were acting arbitrarily or were making decisions on less than adequate information? This awkwardness is exaggerated by tunnel vision, impatience, time pressure, and operating on the basis of untested assumptions. When challenged, professionals will respond with defensive reasoning. They are threatened by the prospect of critically examining their own role and prefer to insist that the fault lies with others. This scenario is commonplace in organizations where failure is unacceptable, where knowing is more important than learning. "Questioning needs to be seen not as a sign of mistrust or as an invasion of privacy, but as a valuable opportunity for learning" (Argyris 1991).

> Support people to believe that they can create what they want, reach for what they truly value, and take personal responsibility for both their vision and existing circumstances. What you believe determines what you perceive as reality. What you believe determines what you feel you can do about it. What you believe determines the exhilaration and joy you get out of life. Beliefs can be changed. The essence of the metanoic shift is the realization within each individual of the extraordinary power of a group committed to a common vision. They believe in the power of visioning, the power of the individual to determine his or her own destiny. They know that through responsible participation they can empower each other and ultimately their institution and society, thereby creating a life that is meaningful and satisfying for everyone (Argyris 1991).

PHYSICIANS AND RESISTANCE TO CHANGE

How physicians see the world and how they act are functions of their underlying beliefs and attitudes. Their training in scientific reductionism and the role they play in society cause physicians to be even more rigid in their adherence to their underlying beliefs and attitudes. This reductionistic view prompts them to see the world in terms that are objective, measured, and quantifiable. They perceive the truth in absolute terms. Little importance is attributed to the qualitative and subjective. This training is reinforced by the need of both patients and physicians to see the physician as absolute authority.

> Attitudes have a kind of inertia. Once set in motion, they will keep going, even in the face of the evidence. To change an attitude requires a considerable amount of work and suffering. The process must begin either in a constantly maintained posture of self-doubt and criticism or else in a painful acknowledgment that what we thought was right all along may not be right after all. Then it proceeds into a state of confusion. This state is quite uncomfortable; we no longer seem to know what is right or wrong or which way to go. But it is a state of openness and therefore of learning and growing. It is only from the quicksand of confusion that we are able to lead to the new and better vision (Peck 1998).

In order to learn, beliefs and attitudes have to be questioned. A level of openness to the opinions of others, a willingness to have your own logic examined by others, and a certain vulnerability that attends admitting that your long-held world-view is incorrect are required. Challenging beliefs and attitudes in effect challenges our own identity. This is particularly difficult for persons whose role is attended by significant positional power. Self-conviction, narcissism, and arrogance begin to color their world view. Change is difficult and challenging work. Laziness and narcissism combine to reinforce the status quo. "We are too lazy to learn and too arrogant to think we need to learn" (Peck 1998).

GROUPS REINFORCE RESISTANCE TO CHANGE

Peck further notes: "Responsibility becomes diffused within groups—so much so that in larger groups it may become non-existent. As groups become larger and larger, their institutions become absolutely faceless. Soulless .... Although there are such phenomena as group identity, group narcissism, and group spirit, there is no way to influence such phenomena except through influencing individual members of the group" (Peck 1998). When physicians are together in a group, underlying attitudes and beliefs are significantly reinforced. The group is a group specifically because those in it share similar beliefs and attitudes. Those who would challenge these shared beliefs challenge the very viability of the group. Groups never change, only individuals change (O'Toole 1995). In the absence of shared and significant external threat, all groups resist change. Any approach to leading and managing change in the physician community cannot be successful if it seeks to manage for group consensus.

THE POWER OF METAPHOR

People learn through metaphor. Through the use of analogy, metaphor allows individuals to see things differently. The use of metaphor can help promote organizational adaptability (Annas 1996). Most of today's healthcare organizations still reflect an industrial model of top-down organizational design. They tend to be traditional command and control organizations in which military and economic metaphors dominate. From the military perspective, there is an emphasis on the physical, seeing control as the key, and a willingness to expend massive resources to ensure dominance. They treat the patient's body as a battlefield with a focus on short-term, single-minded tactical gains. From an economic view, market metaphors dominate. Medical expenditures are losses, mergers and acquisitions with concerns for antitrust become commonplace, and a healthy bottom line replaces a healthy patient as the definition of success. We begin to see medicine in terms of patient satisfaction, ability to pay, profit maximization, entrepreneurship, efficiency, and competition. These organizations are competitive, fragmented, and reactive instead of collaborative, integrated, and proactive.

What would these organizations be like if they adopted an ecology metaphor characterized by words like integrity, tolerance, diversity, renewability, responsibility, community, conservation, sustainability, natural, and limited? They might not focus on short-term gains but rather seek solutions that would preserve a system for their grandchildren. They might emphasize quality over quantity.

A fitness landscape is a useful metaphor that challenges the traditional organizational model of top down command and control (Kaufman 1995). If adaptability is represented by the height of the organization above the existing landscape, the higher you are the better adapted you are for meeting current challenges. As you survey the entire landscape, you come to appreciate that others exist at heights that surpass your own. To achieve greater success, you must climb down your hill in order to ascend another that will allow you reach a higher altitude. This represents the need to leave behind legacy skills and relationships and to deconstruct the existing in order to achieve greater success through the adoption of newer beliefs, attitudes, and behaviors. A part of you has to die in order for you to be reborn. You must possess a willingness to let go of who you are in pursuit of who you can become.

CONCLUSION

The pace and magnitude of change is progressing exponentially (Russell 1998). Adaptability and flexibility are essential to sustainability. The old models of command and control, long-term strategic planning, and demands for certain knowledge as a prerequisite to action do not work. We must acknowledge that we exist within complex adaptive systems and that to sustain we must create learning environments and appreciate how we create our own realities and own future.

Metaphor is an important avenue for communicating new ideas. Adopting an ecological metaphor instead of competitive sports, military, or economic metaphors allows different conclusions to be drawn from viewing the same information. The underlying beliefs and attitudes of the physician community can only be changed if individual physicians bring to the surface their operating assumptions and examine whether they remain valid in light of a changing environment. William James said that the greatest revolution in our generation is the discovery that human beings by changing the inner attitudes of their minds can change the outer aspects of their lives.

NOTES

1. *Edgeware* by Brenda Zimmerman, et al. is a wonderful primer on complexity science and how it applies to the challenges of leading and managing healthcare organizations (Zimmerman and Plsek 1998).
2. The allegory of the tragedy of the commons is presented in Peter Senge's book, *The Fifth Discipline*. This book is a marvelous compendium that should be read several times in order to fully appreciate the wealth of understanding that lies within its covers. In many ways it is the actualization of elements of complexity into an understanding of individual and organizational behavior (Senge 1990).
3. *Complexity* by M. Mitchell Waldrop is a wonderful tour through the evolution of complexity science as it emerged at the Santa Fe Institute. The many principles of complexity science are told through contributions made by physicists, economists, biologists, and computer scientists among others (Waldrop 1992).

4. Margaret Wheatley's book, *Leadership and the New Science* is another easily understood yet elegant presentation of complexity (new) science and its relationship to organizations (Wheatley 1994).

5. Jeffrey Pfeffer's book, *The Human Equation,* is an insightful treatise on the value of teamwork around principles that align incentives. Investing in people is the key to organizational sustainability and provides the one strategic advantage that cannot be duplicated (Pfeffer 1998).

6. *Flight of the Buffalo,* by James Belasco and Ralph Stayer examines how an over-controlling management team interferes with the inherent capacities within the workforce (Belasco and Stayer 1993).

7. Gareth Morgan is a superb teacher who emphasizes that individuals learn through metaphor and store information as narrative. His books, *Images of Organization,* and *Imagin-I-zation,* are very instructive and help develop a better understanding of organizational behavior (Morgan 1997).

8. The Institute for Healthcare Improvement has emphasized action-based change as a way to expedite clinical process improvement. This approach to change is initially very foreign to physicians who are conditioned to view data through the lens of prospective, single-variable, double-blind, randomized controlled studies that produce significant P values and involve a significant N of participants. It is also foreign to the hospital culture that seeks above all else to create change that is acceptable to all and is widely applicable throughout the organization.

9. Peter Senge has published a follow-up book to *The Fifth Discipline* titled, *The Dance of Change.* His experience trying to help develop learning organizations identified significant barriers to its adoption. This text describes ways of reducing those barriers (Senge 1998).

REFERENCES

Argyris, C. 1991. "Teaching Smart People How to Learn." *Harvard Business Review* 69 (3): 99-110.

Belesco, J., and R. Stayer. 1993. *Flight of the Buffalo*. New York: Warner Books.

Kaufman, S. 1993. *At Home in the Universe: The Search for Laws of Self-Organization and Complexity*. New York: Oxford University Press.

Morgan, G. 1997. *Images of Organization*. Thousand Oaks, CA: Sage Publications.

O'Toole, J. 1995. *Leading Change: Overcoming the Ideology of Comfort and the Tyranny of Custom*. San Francisco: Jossey-Bass.

Peck, S. 1998. *People of the Lie: The Hope for Healing Human Evil*. New York: Simon and Schuster.

Pfeffer, J. 1998. *The Human Equation: Building Profits by Putting People First*. Boston, MA: Harvard Business School Press.

Russell, P. 1998. *Waking Up In Time: Finding Inner Peace in Times of Accelerating Change*. Novato, CA: Origin Press.

Senge, P. 1990. *The Fifth Disciple*. New York: Doubleday.

———. 1998. *The Dance of Change: The Challenges of Sustaining Momentum in Learning Organizations*. New York: Currency/Doubleday.

Waldrop, M. M. 1992. *Complexity: the Emerging Science at the Edge of Order and Chaos*. New York: Simon & Schuster.

Wheatley, M. 1994. *Leadership and the New Science Revised: Discovering Order in a Chaotic World*. San Francisco: Berrett-Kohler.

Zimmerman, B., and P. Plsek. 1998. *Edgeware*. Irving, Texas: VHA, Inc.

Chapter Six

LEADERSHIP AND MANAGEMENT: BALANCING INSPIRATION AND PREDICTABILITY

Whenever you see a successful business, someone once made a courageous decision.

Peter Drucker

Success requires three bones—wishbone, backbone, and funnybone.

Kobi Yamada

THE ROLE OF leadership in change management is very important. Although the environment in which physician leaders work presents unique challenges, the tools for success as well as the reasons for failure are no different from nonphysician leaders and, in fact, nonhealthcare leaders.

Are leaders born? Can they be taught? The answer to both questions is yes. Some leadership characteristics are determined genetically and some leadership traits can be taught. What combination of genetic predisposition and social experiences creates a Mother Teresa, a Martin Luther King, Jr., or a John F. Kennedy?

The literature on leadership can guide some thoughtful discussions that will maximize the leadership potential of anyone.

The acid test of leadership is the number and frequency of followers. Without followers, there is no leadership. This chapter will address why some individuals are able to inspire others to follow them and the potential problems that arise when someone believes he or she is a leader, but no one follows.

LEADERSHIP AND MANAGEMENT

The single most important intangible input in the change process is leadership. We have discussed the importance of the mission, values, and vision statements to building a collective culture and identified the important differences between the collective and expert cultures. The most important difference is that expert cultures do not need mission and values statements—only a shared vision. Regardless of whether your change process involves collectives or experts, the constant is the critical role played by leadership.

The noun "leadership" is used often and in many situations. Sometimes the words leadership and management are used interchangeably. For purposes of this book, leadership and management are considered to be separate but complementary dynamics. Excellent managers are usually technically competent, tactically oriented, focused on short-term outcomes, and results driven. By comparison, great leaders are often defined as visionary, charismatic, big-picture focused, and great communicators. The differences between these two style types can be boiled down to the effect they have on others. Leaders, for example, produce *inspired followers*, whereas managers produce *predictable results*.

LEADERSHIP AND HEALTHCARE

Healthcare is overmanaged and underled. In an industry in seemingly constant change, healthcare leaders have become much better at producing predictable results than helping the workforce become the best professionals possible. Often the seduction of the easy-to-measure tangibles such as finances and productivity take preference over the more complicated but equally important intangibles such as pride, commitment, and joy in work. While tangibles are important, long term success is possible only when the tangibles and the intangibles are in balance, that is, when management's predictability and leadership's inspiration are both extant in the same organization. A short phrase may help to emphasize the importance of balancing leadership and management—It takes two wings to fly!

Leadership research points to one important factor—leaders have followers. One tendency is to confuse professional titles with leadership. Titles are bestowed, usually by an employer. Leadership, on the other hand, is earned—and must be re-earned every day. There is no equity in leadership. Each day a leader must earn the right to have followers. *Leaders have followers who commit to achieving a vision by building teams to manage change.*

Why would one person follow another? A follower believes that the leader is going to a place better than what currently exists. The two elements that establish this special connection between leaders and follower are a clear vision of this better place and the ability to communicate the benefits of achieving the vision.

FOUR FUNDAMENTAL LEADERSHIP TRAITS

Warren Bennis, Ph.D. is a premier researcher and writer on the topic of leadership. In an interview in the *Journal of Healthcare Management,* Dr. Bennis discussed the four traits that followers want in their leaders (Johnson 1998): *meaning and direction, trust, hope and optimism, and results.* Dr. Bennis stated: "Effective leaders have to actually provide purpose, enable authentic relationships among their people, have a sense of hardiness themselves, and, finally, have the courage to take risks—basically the capacity to act" (Johnson 1998). Each of these traits is intangible and their existence in leaders is a function of perception. The lesson for leaders is how to anticipate the needs of potential followers in developing these four traits. The answer lies in Bennis' phrase— "The courage to act" (Johnson 1998).

A healthcare leader today needs courage. Any fool can fix yesterday's problems. Courage is required to create and communicate an inspiring vision and produce results that show serious intent. Remember, the *only* antidote to skepticism is results.

Meaning and direction. What can be learned from Bennis' four points? Dr. Bennis puts meaning and direction together. However, meaning and direction represent two different leadership factors. Meaning gives work purpose. Money is a very popular topic in healthcare today. The argument has been made that money is so important because working in healthcare today is so joyless. Humans perform unusual, difficult, and complex tasks for "psychic income." Psychic income is that payoff we receive when we achieve something of importance as defined by our values. How much money do you receive to go to the church of your choice, to play golf, or to visit or care for a loved one? We are constantly doing things that make us feel good or that we enjoy. However, because healthcare has become toxic to professional joy, the loss of psychic income is compensated by an extraordinary interest in financial income. The logic may be as follows: If they are going to treat me like a doormat, at least they are going to pay me a lot of money. The inspiration of a leader should provide a meaning beyond dollars and thus create a psychic income for followers.

In terms of direction, when a person's work is meaningful the person feels comfortable that the future is bright; that is, a clear direction has been defined. People will follow those who are taking them to a better place. A vision is the main ingredient to successfully working within an expert culture, for example, physicians.

Trust. Bennis believes people want to trust their leaders. Trust is the combination of honesty, openness, and reliability—as perceived by the receiver. Once again, perception is important. A group of followers must perceive that the leader is telling the truth (honesty), telling them everything (openness), and most importantly being consistent (reliability). Because followers must see the leader as reliable, several interactions are necessary before trust will be established and subsequently strengthened. Trust cannot be built with one interaction. In fact, trust increases in direct relationship to the frequency of meaningful interactions. Of course, the definition of "meaningful" is the minds of the potential followers.

Hope and optimism. Leaders must produce hope and optimism. While Dr. Bennis does not identify a hierarchy in these four areas, it might be useful to view them that way. For example, change begins with establishment of meaningful work (a mission statement) and a clear direction for the future (a vision statement). When these statements become real in terms of leadership's verbal and behavioral communication strategies, trust is formed. Hope and optimism can easily be the next target for leaders to elicit from followers. The possibility of eliciting hope and optimism without meaning, direction, and trust seems unlikely; or at best short lived. Both hope and optimism can only be engendered when the leader is able to communicate the benefits of vision achievement. People will tolerate great amounts of frustration if the end result is attractive and desirable. The best way to demonstrate that things are improving and that there are reasons to be hopeful and optimistic is to produce results.

Results. Leaders need to produce for their followers. In today's healthcare systems, talking and studying seem to have replaced results. There is some unwritten notion that if we are talking about a problem, we are doing something about it. A wise orthopedic physician in Wisconsin recently said: "Here in Wisconsin, we learned a long time ago that—you don't fatten a cow by weighing it!" The noted leadership guru Tom Peters has said for years to "try it, fix it, do it" and "ready, fire, aim." Positive organizational change is a function of a series of small wins that are tied to a shared vision and supported by a group of followers. People want to work for an organization that is led by someone who says what they are going to do, does it, shares the recognition, and says what they are going to do next. The phrase used in organizational change theory is *positive behavioral contagion*. Positive results are contagious, neutralize the skeptics, and create an infrastructure upon which to build further change. Results also produce consequences such as increased trust, hope, and optimism about the future, that is, all the things Dr. Bennis says followers want. Leaders produce results.

LEADERSHIP AND EFFECTIVE COMMUNICATON

Effective communication is the best way to move from talking to doing. Two guidelines help explain why communication in healthcare is difficult and may result in different messages being received from the messages intended: (1) always talk in the language of the receiver; and (2) always log-in before sending your message.

The language of the receiver. The language of the receiver is determined by motivational influences, status in the organization, degree of the perception of threat, and history with the message giver, that is the degree of trust. For example, the language that excites senior executives may be incomprehensible to those at another layer of the organization.

Executives are motivated by power and achievement, and the people who report to them are usually motivated by affiliation. The words and language patterns used by executives is foreign to the rest of the staff. A common response of American travelers in a foreign land in which they do not speak the language is to talk louder. Like at some auditory threshold, "these foreigners" will understand English! This dynamic is also common in healthcare. Executives seem to believe that at some critical mass of memos, e-mails, or meetings, the receivers of the messages will have a sudden epiphany and all will be clear. Leaders must talk in the language of the receiver. Increasing the volume is not the solution to comprehension.

Log-in before sending your message. The second communication guideline for leading change with all healthcare professionals is to always "log-in." All humans have log-in codes. These codes behave the same way that a log-in code works with a computer. Without the code, you cannot access the computer's brain. Without the human code, you cannot access the human brain. For example, when talking to trustees and financial officers about bond ratings the log-in code is a combination of financial words. The same cluster of words that unlocks the brains and thoughts of those interested in bonds will shut down those interested in quality of care. A leader should form initial comments to highlight the benefits of the listener. Each audience will have a different list of benefits. These benefit lists are the log-in codes for that group. Communication is the bridge between managing change and reacting to change.

LEADERSHIP AND CHANGE

There are three types of change: *evolutionary, autocratic, and managed.* A different leadership style is manifest in each of these change types.

EVOLUTIONARY CHANGE

Evolutionary change is the kind of change that is imbedded in the system. Nothing can be done about evolutionary change except minimize the outcomes. An example of evolutionary change is the aging process. It goes on twenty-four hours a day, seven days a week. We cannot alter the aging process (and stopping it is a bit radical!). However, we can minimize the effects of the aging process with a healthy life style. A similar evolutionary process exists in healthcare—bureaucracy. Bureaucrats seem to multiply at an accelerating rate. A healthcare leader can not slow down his or her own growth. A good leadership style when involved with evolutionary change is to try to minimize damage to the caregivers. The degree that the bureaucratic hoops can be jumped through in the business office, legal department, and executive suite indicates the degree to which caregivers will feel better about leadership.

AUTOCRATIC CHANGE

The autocratic leadership style is not advised except in times of greatest crises. Those who routinely manifest an autocratic leadership style are doomed to fail in the long run. Autocratic behavior reinforces the person who displays it. Because people jump when the autocrat makes a command, the autocrat thinks that the reason for the "quick action." The quick responses they see are nothing more than people displaying the minimum behavior required to make the autocrat go away—then they return to what they were doing before being yelled at. The biggest problem of autocratic change is the long-term effects on the organization. Autocratic leadership *style* always produces passive aggressive behavior. Passive aggressive behavior will always destroy an organization in the long run. As mentioned earlier, passive aggressivity is a silent killer.

MANAGED CHANGE

Managed change is used by effective leaders and is characterized by five stages:

- Create a vision.
- Think small: Divide the vision into strategic imperatives, tactical plans, and individual accountabilities.
- Move fast: Create a set of short-term targets and appropriate accountabilities.
- Evaluate: Design a set of metrics which demonstrate progress in short time periods.
- Celebrate: Showcase the progress and recognize the persons responsible.

Healthcare is a noble and important profession providing one of the most important human needs—caring for the sick and dying. We should celibrate this gift of working in one of the best industries in society.

Why managed change works. Managed change techniques work because effective leaders break down vision-driven tasks into smaller tasks and hold staff accountable for measurable gain. The reason that this leadership style is so effective is not the mechanics, although the mechanics must be in place; these leaders have the ability to maximize the potential of the staff through shared celebration at each measured point of success. They continue to put a high value on psychic income. Failure is usually a function of poor design of the change process, not the quality of the staff performing the tasks.

John Kotter, Ph.D. has an impressive body of research on successful leaders and unsuccessful leaders. His wrote an excellent *Harvard Business Review* article titled: "Why Transformational Efforts Fail" (Kotter 1995). The article lists eight developmental steps to transforming an organization (Figure 6.1). These steps reinforce the notion that effective leaders use the five-part change management process mentioned above.

Kotter's advice is relevant to today's healthcare environment in many ways. The foremost aspect in the failure to transform organizational behavior within expert (i.e., physician) cultures is

Figure 6.1 Eight Steps to Transforming Your Organization

Step 1: Establishing a Sense of Urgency
- Examine market and competitive realities
- Identify and discuss crises, potential crises, or major opportunities

Step 2: Forming a Powerful Guiding Coalition
- Assemble a group with enough power to lead the change effort
- Encourage the group to work together as a team

Step 3: Creating a Vision
- Create a vision to help direct the change effort
- Develop strategies for achieving that vision

Step 4: Communicating the Vision
- Use every vehicle possible to communicate the new vision and strategies
- Teach new behaviors by the example of the guiding coalition

Step 5: Empowering Others to Act on the Vision
- Get rid of obstacles to change
- Change systems or structures that seriously undermine the vision
- Encourage risk taking and nontraditional ideas, activities, and actions

the relationship between establishing a sense of urgency and creating a vision. Too often a crisis precipitates the need to engage a group of physicians. The sense of urgency is real; however, the approach is viewed as crisis management not thoughtful, planned, long-term behavioral change. Experts will behave differently when they understand how they fit into the vision of the future. Urgency without a context is counterproductive. Successful leaders of change build connections between vision and reality.

Figure 6.1 (continued)

Step 6: Planning for and Creating Short-Term Wins
- Plan for visible performance improvements
- Create those improvements
- Recognize and reward employees involved in the improvements

Step 7: Consolidating Improvements and Producing Still More Change
- Use increased credibility to change systems, structures, and policies that don't fit the vision
- Hire, promote, and develop employees who can implement the vision
- Reinvigorate the process with new projects, themes, and change agents

Step 8: Institutionalizing New Approaches
- Articulate the connections between the new behaviors and corporate success
- Develop the means to ensure leadership development and succession

Adapted from Kotter, J. 1995. "Why Transformational Efforts Fail." *Harvard Business Review* (Mar/Apr) p. 61.

Donald N. Sull wrote about this phenomenon in *Why Good Companies Go Bad* (Sull 1999). Sull uses the phrase "active inertia" to describe how executives of failing organizations unleash a flurry of initiatives in response to a threat. He states: "Active inertia is an organization's tendency to follow established patterns of behavior — even in response to dramatic environmental shifts. Stuck in the modes of thinking and working that brought success in the past, market leaders simply accelerate all their tried-and-true activities. In trying to dig themselves out of a hole, they just deepen it" (Sull 1999). Could active inertia explain why so many attempted partnerships with physicians become adversarial? Active inertia needs to be replaced with a new, agreed-upon vision wherein all parties see their self-interest. The lesson from both Kotter and Sull is that a process of change exists that works. However, the nature of organizations is to repeat previous behavior regardless of the need for a fresh, visionary, inclusive approach to creating a new future in which all parties benefit. The ability to create a clear vision, which operates under the principles of a non-zero sum game, is the way to maximize success.

THE FOCUS-FIT-FINISH FORMULA

Expert cultures are lead best when all the parties are clear about the same outcome, know how they fit into successful achievement of the goal, and know when the objective is achieved. Collectives, on the other hand, have a strong interest in the integrity of the group. Sometimes group cohesiveness takes precedence over goal achievement. Leaders understand that in order to achieve a desired outcome with experts they must be clear about "focus-fit-finish." Mistakes are made when group process techniques replace this simple formula. No one can change the motivational patterns of either experts or collectives. The best a leader can do with experts is to accept the behavioral patterns as real and leverage their strengths for the good of the organization.

A common parable provides a lesson that captures the importance of the focus-fit-finish motif with experts. The parable is about the scorpion and the frog. The scorpion wanted to cross the pond but could not swim so he asked the frog to carry him across the pond. The frog did not trust the scorpion and the frog asked the scorpion whether he would be stung. The scorpion responded that stinging the frog would not be in his best interest because that would kill the frog. The frog agrees to carry the scorpion across the pond. Halfway across the pond, the scorpion stings the frog. Before dying the frog asked, "Why did you sting me? Now we will both die." The scorpion replied, "I am a scorpion, I have to sting you—it's my nature!"

The important lesson in this story is that all humans have a unique and special nature. Each of us is motivated differently; we have our own way of thinking and style of relating to others. There is a definite limit to how much we can remold someone. We should not focus on the differences and try to grind them down. Instead, we need to *capitalize* on them. Leaders try to help each person become *more* of what already exists. Very simply: *focus* a clear vision; *fit* the right people into the roles to be successful; and *finish* the tasks that will achieve the vision. Depending on the ethos of the group, you may wish to consider yet another "F" word—*fun*. Celebration is a powerful tool in organizational effectiveness. Whether any fun (i.e., celebration of success) is engaged within an expert culture is the leader's judgment call.

CONCLUSION

Both leadership and management are needed for success in today's healthcare environment, especially when creating physician partnerships. The number of followers defines leadership. Leaders are inspirational and visionary. Managers are able to produce predictable results. The complementary dynamics of successful change are inspired followers and predictable results. Leaders need courage, and all staff, both experts and collectives, want to follow a leader who they believe is taking them to a better place. Courage, a sense of direction, trust, and hope are essential to meaningful change.

The way leaders communicate determines their success. Leaders intuitively "log-in" and always "talk in the language of the receiver." Leaders are able to communicate the vision in ways that inspire commitment and possess an ability to break the vision into doable tasks wherein the participants see their own self-interests. The leader knows that experts are not going to change their personality. They focus on using the strengths of the expert, not trying to change them. Finally, leaders manage change because they focus on the vision, fit the expert to the task, and finish the tasks that fulfill the vision. Leaders may even have fun in celebrating success.

REFERENCES

Johnson, J. A. 1998. "Warren Bennis, Chairman, The Leadership Institute." *Journal of Healthcare Management* 43(4): 293–296.

Kotter, J. 1995. "Why Transformational Efforts Fail." *Harvard Business Review* (Mar/Apr) 73(2): 59, chart 4c.

Sull, D. N. 1999. "Why Good Companies Go Bad." *Harvard Business Review* (July/Aug) 77(4): 42, chart 2c.

Chapter Seven

TRUST: THE
STRATEGIC IMPERATIVE

As we become more civilized we are beginning to emphasize
not the differences that lead to antagonism but the common
impulses and desires which lead to better understanding.

Will Mayo

RUST IS AN essential ingredient in all enduring relationships. Historically, hospitals and their associated medical
staffs have coexisted in somewhat of a "love-hate" relationship. Hospitals do not trust physicians, and physicians do not
trust hospitals. By and large physicians see the hospital as their
workshop, whereas hospital administrators and hospital board
members view the hospital as a community asset. Physicians expect that the hospital will provide them with the tools necessary
for them to carry out their work. Hospital administrators expect
that physicians will readily serve the mission of the organization
(Annison 1998).

Because hospital administrators and physicians view the world through very different lenses, they draw different conclusions when interpreting the same observations. Instead of acknowedging that these different conclusions are the consequence of a different set of operating assumptions, each participant concludes that the other is not trustworthy. Rather than trying to understand the difference in view, the conclusion is made that the other party is merely self-serving. In this chapter we will describe the physician culture, define trust, and outline ways of establishing and building trust between physicians and healthcare organizations.

PHYSICIAN CULTURE[1]

Physician cultural traits include the following:

- emphasis on individual performance;
- respect for personal autonomy;
- competitiveness;
- status conscious;
- unique perception of time;
- difficulty working together;
- personalized decision making; and
- personality clusters within specialties.

Understanding the physician culture highlights the reasons that physicians do not trust other healthcare professionals and even each other.

TEAMWORK: HOW EXPERT CULTURES DIFFER FROM COLLECTIVE CULTURES

Physicians comprise what is referred to as an expert culture (see chapter 4). In expert cultures, an individual's success is a direct consequence of his or her individual skill, knowledge, and ambition. An individual member's contribution to the overall success of the group is defined in terms of performing at his or her isolated best; the whole is the sum of the individual parts. Experts are motivated by accomplishment and power. This focus on individual performance is one of the primary reasons why organizations do not perceive most physicians as good team players. Hospitals, on the other hand, are collective cultures that thrive on teamwork (Atchison 1990). In collective cultures, interdependency is acknowledged and people are motivated by a need for acceptance and recognition. Is there any wonder then why physicians and hospitals respond differently to calls for enhanced teamwork?

PERSONAL AUTONOMY

Whereas today's healthcare environment is demanding that physicians aggregate, physicians are taught to practice as individuals. The entire practice of medicine is focused on the individual doctor-patient relationship. The dominant metaphor is the physician as "captain of the ship," absolutely in command and accountable only to his or her professional standards and ethics. While physicians crave order, they despise authority, particularly in the setting of private medical practice. Physicians who choose to enter into this type of practice are especially covetous of their personal autonomy. Otherwise they might have chosen to work within a formal organizational setting, like academia, the military, or a staff model HMO. An unwillingness to adopt standardized approaches to patient care, ineffective peer review, and a reluctance to subjugate personal interest to the collective good are some examples of the consequences of this overriding value. Frequently the only thing that unites physicians is their mutual commitment to the preservation of individual physician prerogatives.

Physicians may be described as collegial. Collegiality celebrates differences and promotes autonomy and independence. Collaboration, on the other hand, reflects a common culture bound by common vision, values, and business purpose. Collaboration promotes integration and interdependency. Efforts at uniting physicians have often failed because physicians lack a common group identity. If physicians are to become successful and able to assert a collective influence, they will need to accept leadership and demonstrate the ability to follow within the context of a unifying and collaborative identity. It is difficult to predict whether physicians can move beyond the overriding commitment to individual autonomy toward collaboration, where individual success becomes a derivative of collective success.

COMPETITIVENESS

Physicians are highly competitive people (Shell and Klasko 1996). The entire process of becoming a fully trained physician is a competitive one. Physicians compete for admission to medical school, the best residencies, good practice opportunities, and success vis-a-vis their colleagues. When you are competitive, you do not trust others. You play your cards close to your vest. You do not openly reveal your strategies. You do not share knowledge, because knowledge is an advantage.

The formation of a partnership requires negotiation. Having decided to negotiate, you can adopt one of four primary approaches:

1) you can compete—termed win/lose;
2) you can accommodate—termed lose/win;
3) you can collaborate—a form of win/win; or
4) you can compromise—termed lose/lose.

Not surprisingly, studies by Shell and Klasko demonstrate that physicians prefer to compete, that is, play win/lose (Shell and Klasko 1996). The insightful observation in their study is that when confronted with the possibility of losing in a game of win/lose, physicians will default to lose/lose (compromise) rather than win/win (collaboration). Compromise is preferable because in order to collaborate you have to be able to trust, and competitive physicians do not trust each other, let alone outsiders. In effect, although the physician may not get all he or she may want from the negotiation, neither does the other side, and that saves face. The thought that both sides could win with the adoption of a collaborative solution is beyond the physicians' competitive frame of reference (Shell and Klasko 1996).

STATUS CONSCIOUSNESS

Physicians train in a hierarchical environment and therefore are very status conscious. Nowhere is this more evident than on teaching rounds in a hospital. The group may consist of a professor, junior professor, chief resident, senior resident, junior resident, and medical students. Each defers to those of higher status. The ultimate goal is to ascend to the point of highest authority such that those beneath you rarely challenge your judgment. This experience makes it difficult for physicians to relate to others who they perceive to be of a lower status. It reinforces the notion that the physician is " the captain of the ship." They constantly want to direct those around them. Status consciousness is another reason why physicians are often poor team players (Shell and Klasko 1996).

PERCEPTION OF TIME

The manner in which physicians perceive time distinguishes them from hospital administrators. Physicians perceive time in the very near term. To a physician, now means yesterday: Problems are analyzed, judgments are made promptly, and the need for action perceived as immediate. Once physicians make a decision, they want what they need now. A hospital administrator's time is often measured in budget cycles. Decisions are made in a more systematic way with consideration given to the widespread ramifications of the decision. Resources that are allocated to satisfy one need restrict resources that might be available in support of other initiatives. To the physician, all that matters is what his or her patient needs at the moment.

DIFFICULTY WORKING TOGETHER

Physicians have no frame of reference for how to work together. The only time they get together in a setting away from the patient's bedside is at medical staff meetings. The term organized medical staff is an oxymoron. Anyone who has tried to conduct business at a medical staff meeting will appreciate the difficulty in accomplishing anything meaningful. Examine how difficult it is to accomplish peer review and credentialing activities. Any controversy over an issue can be tabled. Physicians manage for consensus and end up finding a solution that is the least objectionable to the most persons. The attempt to create consensus demands that all initiatives be acceptable to all related departments or committees. Any solution that emerges is so watered down that it threatens nobody and is without impact. The overriding consideration at all physician meetings is the preservation of individual autonomy. No collective identity, or formal acknowledgment of leadership roles exist beyond what is ceremonial and representational. No attempt is made to follow and come together around issues of common interest (Bujak 1999).

Physician are individualistic and there is no precedent on which they can appreciate how process design might improve their medical outcomes. Is there any wonder why they cannot adopt a view that would allow for individual success to be a derivative of collective success? Why they are not good "team players" as defined by clear role interdependency? They do not speak with a unified voice. Due to their cultural characteristics, physicians are organizationally impaired.

DECISION MAKING

Physicians tend to make decisions that are personalized, anecdotal, linear, and relate to a very short time frame of reference.
Their training in scientific reductionism conditions them to respond in that way. Deductive reasoning teaches them to think in
linear terms rather than adopting a more systemic perspective.
Lacking significant outcomes data, they are anecdotal and are
disproportionately influenced by their most recent experiences,
tending to repeat what worked the last time. Working within an
expert culture in which accountability is individualized, they
tend to view issues with a personalized frame of reference: how
will this affect me, rather than how will this affect the larger context? Those in expert cultures do not often consider ramifications
beyond their immediate personal needs.

PERSONALITY CLUSTERS WITHIN SPECIALTIES

The medical community has a number of conflicting subsets:
primary care physicians versus specialists, urban versus rural, hospital-based specialists versus non-hospital based-physicians, aca-
demicians versus community practitioners, and age-related behavioral and attitudinal differences that cut across these subsets.

These subsets are further influenced by personality traits that
superimpose themselves on various specialties within the physician community. Surgeons are prone to action. They want to fix
things, now. They want to make quick judgments and move on.
Internists, on the other hand, are trained to think in terms of "rule
outs." They can tell you all the reasons why something will not
work and are unable to acknowledge that a proposal might be
applicable most of the time and therefore be worth adopting.
Pediatricians and family practitioners are more focused on relationships and are particularly sensitive to the feelings and considerations of others. These differences help explain why attempts

to organize physicians meet with such difficulties. Subgroups prioritize their values differently and respond to individual initiatives in ways that uniquely reflect their perspective and their self-interests.

TRUST

In this section we will define trust, explore how trust is first established, describe ways to build trusting relationships, and list specific behaviors that can encourage and maintain a trusting environment. Specific exercises will be discussed that can be used to create an awareness of the need to establish and build trusting relationships.

ELEMENTS OF TRUST

Annison and Bujak (1998) have described seven elements that when together create the feeling of trust taken:

1. *Commitment*: We trust persons who are committed to something more than themselves.
2. *Familiarity*: A willingness to trust is based on how we are treated by others in personal encounters. The more personal contact we have with someone, the more likely we are to appreciate him or her in a way that can engender trust.
3. *Personal responsibility*: We trust people who are willing to take responsibility for their behavior.
4. *Integrity*: Integrity means telling the truth and involves remaining true to yourself and your values in the face of contrary demands.
5. *Consistency*: Consistency is the connection between what we say and what we do. We trust people whose actions are consistent with what they say over time.

6. *Communication:* Open communication is essential to trust. A willingness to discuss sensitive issues often produces surprisingly positive results. When people who disagree talk about their differences, they frequently realize that they have reached different conclusions based on different facts or legitimately different perceptions of the same issue.
7. *Forgiveness and reconciliation:* The willingness to move beyond painful or difficult moments is essential to reconciliation and reestablishing trust.

Trust is the foundation of all successful and enduring relationships. Trust allows people to value the creative possibilities that are inherent in conflict and human diversity (Cooper and Sawarf 1997). People who have mutual trust are free to openly disagree. Their different perspectives can be woven into a tapestry of enriched and divergent viewpoints that extend the range of possible alternatives beyond those available to any one of them alone. The converse is also true. A distrustful environment is worse than a neutral one because the absence of trust predisposes to erroneous assumptions.

ESTABLISHING TRUST

In establishing a trusting relationship, either party can choose to (1) either wait until the other party does something that demonstrates their potential trustworthiness, or (2) be the first to extend trust. The first approach asks the question, What have you done for me lately? It is often motivated by fear of being taken advantage of. The latter approach demonstrates someone who lives more from hope than from fear. Each approach may in fact be its own self-fulfilling prophecy.

Trustworthiness is not decided in the logical brain but rather something that is very quickly and intuitively felt in the limbic brain (Cooper and Sawarf 1997). The limbic brain, which operates approximately 80,000 times faster than the logical cerebral cortex, almost instantaneously synthesizes verbal and nonverbal cues into a subjective assessment of another individual's trustworthiness and believability. It is easier to begin to build a trusting relationship by paying attention to ones intuitive self rather than trying to logically judge, interpret, weigh, and measure the words and actions of others.[2]

Alignment of interests can be difficult when people differ in their beliefs, attitudes, needs, and perceptions. Trust can be established by appreciating the differing perspectives of other parties through empathic listening. As we have seen, however, physicians and hospital administrators have very different perspectives. In interpreting the same data set, they often arrive at different conclusions. Rather than acknowledging and appreciating that different frames of reference reflect differing assumptions, both parties interpret these differences as reflecting different values and motives and conclude that the other cannot be trusted.

A trusting relationship can be established in a number of ways:[3]

- create common vision or goals;
- define shared principles;
- identify a common enemy;
- clarify benefits that can result from collaboration;
- list consequences of failing to cooperate;
- state what you can contribute if barriers to cooperation are removed;
- focus on similarities and not differences;
- identify early wins that can create momentum; and
- listen and identify with the needs and aspirations of your potential partner.

CREATING COMMON VISION OR GOALS

The primary responsibility of leadership is to author, communicate, and promote organizational vision (Kotter 1996). Differing degrees of commitment to new behaviors that reflect the strength of the underlying belief are required. Persons who are committed are willing to break the rules in pursuit of their goals. Those who enroll in new behaviors work within the rules to achieve the desired goals. Beneath these levels of strength of belief are varying degrees of compliance. What separates the committed and enrolled from the compliant is that the former own the vision, whereas the latter accept another's vision. Organizational success therefore reflects the degree to which the organizational vision and the individual participant's vision are consistent and mutually reinforcing. The role of leadership is to formulate and articulate the vision and to mold the organizational culture around shared purpose and values. It is the strength of those intangibles that predict organizational success or failure. As Napoleon has said, "there is no amount of money that you could pay someone that would cause them to lay down their life for you, something they would gladly do for a piece of yellow ribbon" (Waldrop 1996).

Vision versus mission. Vision is distinct from mission. Hospital people often assume that physicians must share their mission. In fact, the words mission, vision, and values have become an alliteration of sorts. They are often used in a string without due consideration for their differences. Successful partnerships must share the same goals or vision. Each participant must see that the vision satisfies his or her individual needs. However, each participant may have a separate mission.

Must physicians share the mission of the healthcare organization? "Serving the healthcare needs of the community" is a component of the mission statement of almost every healthcare organization. If that were the goal of a physician, he or she would work for the local health department or a primary religious-based organization. If the physician seeks to be a competent caregiver, successful business person, spouse, and parent and can see that those objectives can be met within the context of an organizational vision, they can be a committed partner independent of the issues that characterize the mission of the organization.

Vision and leadership. Vision is the job of leadership. Unfortunately, physicians seem unable to lead other physicians (Bujak 1999). While physicians are quick to express their individual opinion, they are reluctant to speak on behalf of their colleagues, because they would resent anyone else presuming to speak for them. Physicians who presume to lead are summarily rejected. In essence, a culture that emphasizes individual autonomy responds with a "who died and left you boss" attitude towards those who would articulate for change.[4] This attitude is reinforced when physicians are present in groups. Groups do not change, only individuals change. The majority will always act to defend the status quo. The current behaviors of a group are manifestations of their shared underlying beliefs and attitudes. An individual must be willing to change underlying beliefs and attitudes in order to change behavior. Those who would articulate for change therefore challenge the group where it is most vulnerable—at the level of their shared assumptions, beliefs, and attitudes, the very glue that binds them together. To acknowledge the rectitude of new ideas is to deny the validity of the shared beliefs and therefore to challenge the very viability of the group (O'Toole 1995).

The power of vision. Individuals lead through the power of vision. "In the absence of a great dream, pettiness prevails" (Kofman and Senge 1993). Since physicians appear to be unable to acknowledge leadership from within, the hospital or health system CEO, in our view, is the one person capable of uniting the provider community in the service of a shared vision. He or she represents a source of necessary capital and can reflect values that are unencumbered by the needs to satisfy for-profit ventures. An organization-physician interdependency is present that further provides a springboard for forming new relationships. For this to occur, hospital boards must fully support their CEO. As noted above, promoting change will cause the majority of physicians to complain and resist. Without unequivocal board support, a CEO seeking to organize the physician community would certainly encounter a career limiting opportunity.

To be successful at organizing the provider community, the CEO must be willing to be pluralistic in his or her response, let go of the presumed need to create consensus among the physicians, and avoid defining success in terms of winning. The metric that defines winning is cast in terms of the rules of the current game and amounts to achieving more points than your opponent. Success can be achieved without someone else losing and can occur because you are willing to change the rules and play a different game. Enemies do not have to be created in order to be successful; those same enemies may be your collaborators in the future.

DEFINE SHARED PRINCIPLES OR VALUES

The values that will define the group must be clarified and prioritized. Through answering "what if" questions and by responding to potential future scenarios, leaders can more clearly communicate the principles that will guide decision making. Equally important is the need to agree upon what metric or metrics will define success. In this way members of the organization can fully appreciate the what and why of the new enterprise and fully understand how difficult judgments are made in pursuit of the organizational vision.

Individual hierarchy of values. Time needs to be spent understanding and prioritizing each other's values (Reece 1999). Everyone has a hierarchy of values that prioritizes his or her commitments. Although there are many different values, only a handful of behaviors in fact represent the manifestations of many different underlying values. For example, if one person prioritizes honesty and another integrity, both of these values are served by a commitment to truthfulness. Once you can identify a cluster of behaviors that reflect the majority of expressed values, you can agree to codes of behaviors that will come to define the organizational culture and reflect mutual commitment. Through the interpretation of expressed behaviors people judge the underlying motivations and beliefs of others. Do not listen to what they say, watch what they do.

Difference between personal values and what a person values. People often fail to understand the difference between personal values and what a person values. Personal values may include honesty, truthfulness, respect, etc. To the extent that partnerships will be successful, personal values must be held in common, or the participants will self-select out of the group. From an organizational perspective, what is valued might be financial success, caring for the poor, technical expertise, or other ways to define core competencies. The hierarchy of organizational values is defined by how the organization prioritizes resource allocations. Because individuals prioritize organizational values differently, multiple ventures are possible if not necessary in order to segment potential partners around different organizational values. Initiatives in one joint venture may have totally different objectives than those of another based on different organizational priorities.

IDENTIFY A COMMON ENEMY

Identifying a common enemy provides a shared negative vision. To organize physicians into a collective and collaborative partnership, leaders must provide both a positive vision and a negative vision. The value of negative vision lies in its ability to galvanize and motivate for immediate action. A negative vision requires immediate action or else suffer the loss of something valuable. Beware, however, a negative vision is never sustaining. Responding to a negative vision will reduce the intensity of threat, thereby reducing the motivation to act. A stop and start response is produced and action only intensifies when the intensity of threat returns to a threshold level. Only positive vision can sustain action over time. Unfortunately, positive vision is something that many persons can wait until tomorrow to pursue, hence the value of a negative vision.

CLARIFY COLLABORATION BENEFITS

Presenting the immediate tangible and intangible benefits that can result from partnering provides a logical quid pro quo that supports the deliverables that will result if the parties agree to collaborate. Ideally, these benefits will result from successfully pursuing the positive vision.

THE CONSEQUENCES OF FAILING TO COOPERATE

Listing the consequences of a failure to cooperate presents the downside of a decision to refuse to partner, and reinforces the negative vision.

STATE CONTRIBUTIONS IF BARRIERS TO COOPERATION ARE REMOVED

Specifying deliverables valued by your potential partner that you can provide immediately if they agree to collaborate furthers a trusting relationship. It may be viewed as analogous to a signing bonus. Rather than focusing on the long-term value that will attend pursuit of the positive vision, it identifies short-term benefits that can be immediately realized.

FOCUS ON SIMILARITIES AND NOT DIFFERENCES

The way to begin this journey is to focus on areas of agreement, not on areas of disagreement. By acknowledging interdependence and focusing on areas of shared agreement, the group can identify initiatives that all would agree are valuable to pursue because they would be in everyone's best interests. Starting at points of agreement allows for joint action, demonstrates trustworthiness, and prevents the new enterprise from getting bogged down in attempts to convince others of the rectitude of their position in areas that attend disagreements.

IDENTIFY EARLY WINS THAT CAN CREATE MOMENTUM

Choosing pilot projects that are meaningful, measurable, and achievable within a short period of time allows the group to achieve successes that deliver hope, trust, and positive momentum. Success reinforces the belief that together they can coauthor their future and from this beginning establish an infrastructure upon which they can build confidence in their relationship and a sense of mutual commitment and shared purpose. Thinking small and building momentum upon many small successes allows the parties to achieve a trusting relationship.[5]

IDENTIFY WITH THE NEEDS OF YOUR POTENTIAL PARTNER

Building a partnership is not the same as doing a deal. A mutual commitment has to be foremost to the success of the relationship. Seek to listen and identify the needs of the other party. Selfish wins at the other's expense might provide short-term advantage for one of the parties, but in destroying trust, it erodes the relationship and promotes dissolution of the partnership. .

Successful partnerships demand that preservation of the relationship be paramount. For that to occur, each party must primarily concern itself with understanding and trying to meet the needs of the other. To this end it is useful to appreciate the distinction between discussion and dialog (Senge 1990). Discussion is a convergent process designed to arrive at a conclusion wherein each advocates for his or her viewpoint and consensus judgment tries to fashion the best available solution at the moment. Dialog is a divergent process that seeks to extend the range of possibilities and demands both advocacy and inquiry. Questioning must be seen as an opportunity to learn and not as a challenge to individual competence. It requires an atmosphere of trust and vulnerability. In order to change your mind you have to alter your beliefs and attitudes and admit that you have been wrong. You need to move through a state of confusion on the way to learning and becoming. Applying competitive metaphors as the framework for defining success will inhibit the necessary curiosity and wonder that supports growth and adaptability.

BEHAVIORS THAT INCREASE TRUST

- Involve others in the process.
- Share information.
- Be proactive. Own your contribution to the present situation.
- Seek to try and meet *their* needs.
- Clarify how changes will affect them.
- Create clear expectations.
- Use data and not anecdote.
- Continue to emphasize common goals and objectives.
- Focus on the future and not the past.
- Keep everyone informed.
- Demonstrate your commitment with action.

Involving others in the process is important because people tend to support that which they help to create. People resent being changed, but they will change if they understand and desire the change and control the process. Sharing information promotes a sense of participation and allows people to feel acknowledged and respected. People want to be "in the know."

Being proactive in change means owning your contribution to the present circumstances and not necessarily being aggressively reactive.[6] Your own behavior is all that you can control. (Fritz 1999). Posturing with an attitude of "if only" and wishing or demanding that others change disempowers you from being a part of the solution and reinforces the viewpoint of a victim.

Clarifying expectations and specifically illustrating how proposed changes are likely to affect the participants is important. People may presume that others will imagine things exactly as they do, because they fail to clearly appreciate the others' operating assumptions and specific interpretations. Physicians and healthcare administrators view the world very differently, and it is exceedingly risky to assume anything without being certain. As Stephen Covey writes, it is important first to understand and then to be understood (Covey 1994).

It is important to reemphasize the importance of keeping everyone informed, and to communicate in the language of the receiver. It is essential to focus on the primary purpose of the partnership and to be consistent in applying the principles that guide decision making. Finally, it is imperative to focus on where you are going and not get caught up in rehashing the past. Complaining and scapegoating are of no value.

ADDITIONAL ACTIVITIES THAT CONTRIBUTE TO SUCCESSFUL COLLABORATION

In collaborative activities you increase trust by:

- establishing mutually agreeable objectives;
- generating scenarios;
- defining mutually agreeable measures;
- creating a time frame;
- assigning accountabilities; and
- discussing what constitutes success and failure.

Too often physicians and healthcare organizations rush to structure a collaborative effort without having spent enough time clarifying the objectives and how they are to be met and measured. Time needs to be spent answering "what if" questions that test clarity of purpose and the values that will guide decision making. Without a time frame and clear accountabilities, good ideas remain a dream and never approximate reality. Clarifying objectives and metrics becomes the basis for defining success and failure. People should value what they measure. They must also measure what they value.

Trust will constantly be challenged by new debates, unfamiliar ground, new expectations and new roles, and by the growing complexity and pressures resulting from the compression of time and space. Without clarity of purpose and shared values, there is no compass that will help to more closely approximate the vision in a rapidly changing world (Annison 1998).

EXERCISES THAT BUILD TRUST

A number of exercises exist that can help build trust. Among these are increased socializing; an exercise called Cover Story, Secret Story, Sacred Story; and formal search conferences.

INCREASING OPPORTUNITIES TO SOCIALIZE

Familiarity facilitates trusting relationships. Any opportunity to socialize has potential for building trust. A retreat is one example of how uninterrupted time together in neutral settings divorced from usual roles can create understandings and friendships not possible in the structured and more narrowly defined professional environment. One of the unfortunate consequences of the increasing time pressures felt by healthcare professionals is the disappearance of socializing. The doctor's lounge, once a beehive for social and professional discussions, now stands empty. Physicians hardly engage their colleagues except in a professional setting.

COVER STORY, SECRET STORY, SACRED STORY

This exercise allows interdependent groups to appreciate what elements they have in common. Individuals often focus on issues that divide them and never realize how much potentially unites them. The exercise is called Cover Story, Secret Story, Sacred Story.[7]

1. *Cover story.* Each constituency in the meeting writes and shares its description of a cover story that would characterize their organization in a way that has maximum appeal to an unfamiliar audience. Imagine how you would like to be portrayed in a featured newspaper article, or how you would present yourself when trying to recruit persons of importance. It is a public relation fantasy about the organization—the most preferred public image.
2. *Secret story.* Next each group describes the organization's secret story; or what really goes on in the organization. This is what we like to say happens, but let me tell you how it really is. This is an opportunity for catharsis and expression of resentments, animosities, frustrations, and anger. The organization's warts and pimples are displayed for everyone to see.
3. *Sacred story.* Finally, each group describes its sacred story. This defines how each group would really like the organization to be: what they really care about; how it affords a place for self-actualization; where they find meaning and purpose; what values are important; and how people should conduct themselves. What invariably emerges are descriptions that are at least 85 percent concordant. It opens an

opportunity to see that others with whom you perceive yourself to be in conflict actually share the same aspirations and values that you do. From the common elements of the sacred stories, areas of agreement can be identified. Because these elements are manifestations that everyone can agree would be of significant value, they become opportunities to jointly build successes and create a sense of optimism, hope, trust, and positive momentum. Through shared action in a shared culture can be forged and solid relationships established.

SEARCH CONFERENCES

Search conferences or facilitated future search retreats provide a very successful way to achieve collective identity and shared commitment towards creating a mutually desired future state (Weisbord and Janoff 2000). The basic elements of the conference include exercises that allow the participants to appreciate that they are affected by and share the same history and environment. A more integrated and systemic view of their interrelationships is acquired and they see how interdependent they are. They describe the current dynamic forces that are transforming their environment and predict the future if those forces are allowed to proceed uninfluenced by a proactive response. That projected future is then contrasted to their own idealized future.

They leave outside the discussion areas of disagreement, and from the elements of their idealized futures that they hold in common, identify specific projects to help create their shared idealized future state. The action plans are very specific with identified expectations and accountabilities, resources, and time lines. A sequence of small successes is built that establishes a sense of growing trust and mutual concern. Solutions lie within the collective wisdom of the group. The entire group is interdependent and responsible for making choices to create a shared and more desirable future. The emphasis is on doing things that are valuable, easy, and measurable.

CONCLUSION

All successful partnerships are based on trust and mutual respect and united by shared vision and values. By following the principles outlined in this chapter, a foundation of trust can be established and enhanced, and an environment of dialog, learning, and growth can be nurtured. Partnering with physicians demands that all participants understand the operating assumptions, beliefs, and attitudes that underlie other's behaviors. Physician culture and the hospital culture are different, and when hospital persons speak about teamwork, it means something very different from the way physicians understand the meaning of the word. Because the behaviors are different, each party concludes the other is not trustworthy, when in fact each is behaving in a way consistent with their own meaning.

We propose that only the CEO of not-for-profit healthcare organizations can organize the physician community, or at least that segment of the community that can see its personal values being enhanced through the joint pursuit of an encompassing vision. For the CEO to be successful in this role, he or she must understand physician culture, have full and unconditional support of the board, and be willing to accept criticism from other segments of the physician community. Success will demand a willingness to forge pluralistic solutions. In many ways a sailing metaphor is useful. Although you cannot control the wind or the current, how you trim the boat and set the tiller will get you closer to your destination, or at least prevent you from being taken further away. When the journey and the destination are the same, the destination is not that critical. You cannot be vested in the literalness of your vision, rather in the qualities that attend that imagined future state.

NOTES

1. Shell and Klasko have written an excellent article describing the behavioral characteristics of physicians. Their research has documented that when physicians confront the probabilities of losing in a game of win/lose, they default to lose/lose or compromise (Shell 1996).
2. Robert Cooper's book on emotional EQ contains a discussion on the neurophysiological basis of trust (Cooper 1997).
3. Ed O'Connor has developed much of the material summarized in the discussion on building trust. Dr. O'Connor is a faculty member of the American College of Physician Executives.
4. James O'Toole's book, *Leading Change: The Argument for Values-Based Leadership*, has had a significant impact on our understanding of group resistance to change. The ideas presented here are adapted from this book, which should be required reading for all who would presume to influence physician behavior (O"Toole 1995).
5. Tom Atchison has successfully applied this approach to transforming culture. His book, *Turning Healthcare Leadership Around*, remains a current and immensely valuable resource (Atchison 1990).
6. The thoughts on personal mastery are from Peter Senge's book, *The Fifth Discipline*, (Senge 1990) and they are further developed in Robert Fritz's book, *The Path of Least Resistance* (Fritz 1989).
7. Birute Regine introduced the exercise called Cover story, Secret story, Sacred story. It is a very useful way to help groups focus on points of agreement.

REFERENCES

Annison, M. J. and J. S. Bujak. 1998. *Trust Matters: How Doctors, Board Members and Health Care Executives Can Work Together Effectively.* La Jolla, CA: Medical Leadership Forum of the Governance Institute.

Atchison, T. A. 1990. *Turning Healthcare Leadership Around: Cultivating Inspired, Empowered, and Loyal Followers.* San Francisco: Jossey-Bass.

Bujak, J. S. 1999. "Culture in Chaos: The Need for Leadership and Followership in Medicine." *Physician Executive* (May/Jun) 25(3): 17–24.

Cooper, R. K., and A. Sawarf. 1997. *Executive EQ: Emotional Intelligence in Leadership and Organization.* New York: Grossett Putnam.

Covey, S., A. R. Merrill, and R. R. Merrill. 1994. *First Things First: To Live, to Love, to Learn, to Leave a Legacy.* New York: Simon and Schuster.

Fritz, R. 1999. *The Path of Least Resistance for Managers: Designing Organizations to Succeed.* San Francisco: Berrett-Koehler.

Kofman, F., and P. Senge. 1993. "Communities of Commitment: The Heart of Learning Organizations." *Organizational Dynamics* 22(5).

Kotter, J. 1996. *Leading Change.* Boston: Harvard Business School Press.

O'Toole, J. 1995. *Leading Change: Overcoming the Ideology of Comfort and Tyranny of Custom.* San Francisco: Jossey-Bass.

Reece, R. L. 1999. "Satisfying Values—Yours and Theirs: A Talk With Manny Elkind." *Physician Executive* 25(6): 18–24.

Senge, P. 1990. *The Fifth Disciple.* New York: Doubleday.

Shell, G. R., and S. K. Klasko. 1996. "Negotiating: Biases Physicians Bring to the Table." *Physician Executive* 22(12): 4–7.

Waldrop, M. M. 1996. "The Trillion-Dollar Vision of Dee Hock." *Fast Company* (Oct) (5) 75.

Weisbord, M. R., and S. Janoff. 2000. *Future Search: An Action Guide to Finding Common Ground in Organizations and Communities.* San Francisco: Berrett-Koehler.

Chapter Eight

YOU ARE WHAT
YOU MEASURE

The greatest thing in this world is not so much where we
stand, as in what direction we are moving.

Goethe

You have brains in your head, and feet in your shoes. You can
steer yourself any direction you choose.

Dr. Seuss

YOU CANNOT MANAGE what you cannot measure. The
use of data is critical to any managed change process.
The role of leadership is to make certain that whatever
is measured is relevant and meaningful to all those responsible
for change.

Measurement is data. Evaluation is judgment. For example,
if someone said, "The board is three feet," that is a measurement.
If someone said, "The board is too short," that is a judgment.
In healthcare this is an important difference because measurement typically involves some use of instrumentation. Evaluation

is the process of assigning value to the scores resulting from the data collection instrument. The term assessment is a common synonym for evaluation. Assessment means that a "yard stick" has been placed against some measures. Collection of data by itself has no impact on change. In fact, collecting data through surveys or other devices and not using the results for positive change can be very frustrating to those surveyed. Healthcare history indicates there are instances where data are collected but the results were shelved. This is very counterproductive and demotivating. Change is possible, and even likely, when the data are viewed as valid and held up to some predetermined standard and interventions are seen as data based.

Both measurement and evaluation are important parts of the managed change process. Managing change is a sequence of procedures that begins with an understanding of the current condition and a clear picture (vision) of the desired condition. Measurement and evaluation allow for a gap analysis of the distance between the current condition and the desired condition. During any managed change process, measurement is used whenever actual tests are used. These tests can be quantitative (i.e., paper and pencil survey instruments) or qualitative (i.e., structured interviews or focus groups). Evaluation is used whenever leadership makes a decision concerning the adequacy of the measures to either establish a baseline for change or highlight the degree of progress from the current condition to the desired state.

MEASUREMENT AND EVALUATION OF THE INTANGIBLES

Evaluation of the intangibles that underlie organizational success in healthcare takes the form of subjective judgment. Countless value judgements are made within all healthcare organizations daily. A large number of problems are created when subjective judgments replace valid data, especially when trying to engage physicians in a change process. The first problem is validity. Is the evaluation true? The second problem is reliability. Can the conclusion be repeated across relevant groups? For example, statements by senior leadership such as "The physicians are unhappy" have no value to a managed change process. The absence of any measurable data from a representative sample makes it impossible to determine what to change. For example:

- Which physicians are unhappy?
- Is it all physicians?
- Is the unhappiness equal among all physicians?
- What are the physicians unhappy about?
- Is the source of their unhappiness something the healthcare organization can do something about?
- Is the source of their unhappiness a function of external forces such as medical macroeconomics?

Image for a minute the same subjective thinking being used in finance. What if the CFO presented a report that began: "We made a lot of money this month." Someone might ask "How much?" The CFO responds "The amount was really big!" The CFO continues, "We did not spend as much as we made, therefore we have a bunch of money left over!" Subjective judgments would never be tolerated in the tangible area of finance. However, when attempting change with the most complicated aspect of healthcare, that is, human behavior, we are amazingly unscientific and noncritical.

MOTIVATIONAL INFLUENCES

Perceptual alignment is the first critical step to successful change management, and motivation is the second. An interesting relationship exists between perception and motivation. Perception equals reality—all humans are 100 percent motivated 100 percent of the time. Motivation cannot be increased or decreased; however, it can be unleashed, directed, or suppressed. We view the world according to our experiences, which determine the direction of the motivation, which drives behavior. Motivation is directed toward those behaviors that are the most meaningful. Meaning is a function of how we view the world. Change management experts use multiple techniques to assess the ways perception affects motivation. Chapter 3 discusses the main motivational influences.

Braskamp and Maehr (1986) make a scholarly presentation on the importance of collecting baseline data about motivational influences. They posit that adult professionals choose to personally invest time and energy in those behaviors that are most consistent with their internal motivational influences. They highlighted four key influences to motivation: recognition, accomplishment, power, and affiliation. In *Turning Healthcare Leadership Around* (Atchison 1990, p. 33–36), these variables are defined and described in the context of the healthcare industry.

Recognition. Some workers crave attention. They continually seek feedback on the quality of their work from their bosses and colleagues. They want to be seen as high-producing winners. They enjoy seeing their names in print, winning awards, and receiving public recognition at special events. For these workers, the emphasis is on external reinforcement for good work through verbal and written plaudits, awards, perks, supplemental benefits, and merit and salary increases.

Accomplishment. Some employees are motivated by productivity, doing the job right, and exploring new opportunities. They are in their offices by 7:30 a.m. and race through project after project. They are eager to get involved in new ventures in the hope of achieving even greater success. Anchored to their desks, these workers rarely take time out for lunch or routine conversation.

Power. Some staff members just want to win. They enjoy going head-to-head with the president of the medical staff, the chairperson of the city planning council, or anyone else. Instead of feeling intimidated by escalating competition from neighboring hospitals, they are exhilarated by it. Their professional life is driven by competition, conflict, and the quest for power.

Affiliation. Finally, some employees want to create a family feeling among their staff members. They invest at least one-third of their day building an atmosphere of trust and camaraderie among their employees. Birthdays, anniversaries, graduations, and births are celebrated with lunches and receptions. When an employee has a personal or family problem, they take time to talk it through and suggest solutions. Their professional life is driven by a desire to respect their employees and to treat them as part of the hospital family.

RELATIONSHIP BETWEEN RECOGNITION AND ACCOMPLISHMENT

The relative importance of the two motivational influences of recognition and accomplishment determine whether a person or group is externally or internally motivated. When recognition dominates accomplishment, the change methodology needs to focus on external rewards. The use of a more linear, management-by-objectives (MBO)-type approach will succeed. Change management interventions with persons and groups who rate accomplishment highly are most successful when the participants are engaged in decisions about goals and deadlines and the ways to achieve those goals are left up to the individuals. Linear and highly structured change methods frustrate high achievement individuals and in fact can run counter to success. Likewise, unstructured interventions with no clear path or end-product rewards will frustrate those with high-recognition needs.

RELATIONSHIP BETWEEN POWER AND AFFILIATION

The relationship between power and affiliation determines the way individuals will behave in groups. When power has more motivational influence than affiliation, the individual or group will be characterized as competitive and prone to conflict. Individuals are motivated by the desire to win rather than what is best for the group. Change management interventions with individuals motivated by power can be very difficult. The challenge for the change leader is to engage such individuals' energy and need to win. This challenge is further complicated if the power-motivated individual is influenced greatly by recognition. Typically, this motivational pattern performs better in a sales organization than in healthcare.

Affiliation-influenced individuals perform best in groups. The need to be with, around, and supported by others is their *raison d'être*. Loyalty and caring for others are the most common descriptors of these individuals. Change management strategies must include a great deal of group process work. The need to be assured and supported can be greater than the need to finish a task. If these individuals have a high need for external recognition, additional problems may arise. High-affiliation and high-recognition motivational patterns are very common in healthcare, especially in direct care providers. Interventions that are successful with high achievers who may also have high power needs (e.g., senior executives and physician leaders) will not work with those with high affiliation and recognition needs.

MOTIVATION AND PERCEPTION DATA

Data about motivation and perception should be gathered at the beginning of any structured change process. We all view the data through our own eyes and our motivational influences are different. Thus, the only way to match interventions with human complexity is to know the degree of perceptual alignment and the main motivational influences. Too often healthcare leaders attempt to manage change without any specific data about the individuals involved in the process. For example, to increase patient and other customer satisfaction scores, a healthcare leader may purchase a program that contains a series of training modules and expect everyone to attend these modules—only to be confronted by unwilling participants. One-size-fits-all, externally driven solutions are not effective change management interventions. In fact, such solutions can erode the very behavior the organization is trying to achieve.

FORMATIVE AND SUMMATIVE EVALUATION

Evaluations must be formed and summarized to move the change process along. Formative evaluations start with periodic data collection. The data are interpreted to promote adjustments in the change process. Formative evaluations ask the following questions:

- How are we doing?
- What is working best?
- What needs to be changed?
- Should any of the interventions be stopped?
- Have we achieved any unintended positive or negative consequences?

Formative evaluations are the basis of all quality improvement techniques.

Summative evaluation results in a conclusion. Summative techniques ask questions such as:

- Did we achieve what we said we would achieve?
- Did we do it in the predicted amount of time?
- Did we do it within budget?

Most summative questions can be answered yes or no.

The behavioral impact of these two types of evaluation is important. Formative evaluations open dialog and promote new learning. Those involved in a change process that focuses on formative data are much more open because the data are simply indicators of what needs to be "fixed." Summative evaluation techniques tend to shut down the behavior of those involved in the change process. Data that are used to summarize the process imply that a good or bad decision will be made. Some person or group will be assigned the blame for the failures. Summative evaluations are used most often with budgets, building projects, clinical paths, and other linear processes. Summative evaluations predictably result in defensiveness and rationalizations. For these reasons, the degree that data are viewed as formative (not summative) will help in maintaining a managed change process. If, on the other hand, data are seen as potential punishers, resistance to change and the creation of a climate of blame will result.

BENCHMARKING FOR DISCOVERY/ IMPROVEMENT

Leaders manage ongoing change through a variety of techniques. Benchmarking seems to be the one technique that has the greatest potency for the longest period of time. This process became popular during the total quality management/continuous quality improvement (TQM/CQI) era in the late 1980's.

Benchmarking is the process of targeting an improvement goal and then locating someone who has already completed the goal successfully. A number of databases exist that are public or available for a fee. Some benefits of locating outside benchmarks are the assumed objectivity of the data and the size of the databases. The weaknesses of outside benchmarks are that the selected database may not match the local population (i.e., it may not be valid), and local staff has a tendency to discount outside benchmarks because: "they don't understand how unique we are!"

INTERNAL BENCHMARKS

The alternative to identifying an outside database is to use internal processes. Within any healthcare organization some departments, units of departments, individual staff, and physicians display desired behaviors at a higher level than most. The internal process of benchmarking is one wherein "best practices" and/or "high performers" are identified. These two techniques can be used independently or in tandem. The way to identify both best practices and high performers is the same. In fact, most of the time when one identifies the high performers, the best practices turn out to be what they do.

CREATING HIGH PERFORMERS

Some people were simply born to be high performers—no matter what the work environment they will always be highly motivated and productive employees. However, high performers can also be created if your work environment fosters the right behaviors. The following steps describe a way to begin developing such an environment within your organization.

1. Bring together the executive team with a meeting facilitator. Each member of the team considers the group of people with whom they work and writes down the names of three to five people who are high performers—their most highly motivated, creative and productive staff, regardless of position or title.
2. Have the facilitator read off the names on each list. In theory, if you have ten senior managers participating in the meeting, you should have 30 to 50 names; however, this is rarely the case. More often, you have at least five individuals whose names appear on more than half the lists. These people are your organization's highest performers. These high

performers should serve as your organization's think tank for identifying ways to increase performance, pride, motivation, and other internal satisfiers. This group should come together once a month for three or four months, then once a quarter after that.

3. Determine what behaviors your high performers have in common. These behaviors will vary from organization to organization, but may include improving processes or volunteering for special projects. Once these high-performing behaviors are identified, incorporate them into your training and education programs, as well as your criteria for promotions, raises, and bonuses. Current high performers will be rewarded and mid-performers will be encouraged to adopt the behaviors.

4. The executive team should identify the low performers — those who do not contribute at all to the success of the organization. Many find this difficult, not because they cannot think of anyone, but because they do not want to name names; however, this is a vital part of this process. Once again, the facilitator reads off the names on each list, and once again, you will find that a handful of people will appear on many of the lists.

5. Determine the common traits of your low performers. These will also vary, but may include such behaviors as missing deadlines or refusing to assist others. Introduce new human resources policies and educational programs designed to eliminate those behaviors, and use them to address the problems of your low performers and train new employees.

By systematically nurturing high performers and decreasing organizational tolerance for low performers, you reinforce those internally motivated people who are producing satisfied customers. This results in a work environment that promotes internal employee satisfaction and, therefore, increased customer satisfaction.

PHYSICIANS AND MEASUREMENT

Physicians function within the boundaries and dynamics of the expert culture. Experts are reluctant to change any behavior simply on the basis of someone's suggestion. Therefore, the way data are collected, the validity of the instruments used to collect data, and the appropriateness of the results to the physician's practice are important lessons concerning physicians and measurement. In fact, without clear evidence that an alternative behavior is superior in one or more ways, physicians will continue to display the behaviors that made them successful. Physician training is based on the scientific method. Double blind, single variable experiments are a common and comfortable methodology for physicians. The results of such research are considered seriously by physicians. Another key factor in the acceptability of any data is the database against which a physician group is compared. For example, medical school faculty must be compared to other teaching facilities of their stature. Community hospital physicians need to know that the comparison database reflects their needs. Subspecialties want to be compared with a database comprised of their specialty peers. Surgeons will not accept as valid data collected on family practice doctors.

DISCERNING PERCEPTION ALIGNMENT

Chapter 3 discusses the role perception plays in controlling behavior. Data about the way physicians perceive the organization are a necessary prerequisite to change management with physicians. The methodology for data collection must comply with the principles detailed in the previous paragraph, that is, validity, reliability, subclassification by specialty, and comparison to a

Table 8.1 Physician Survey

Question	Strongly Agree	Agree	Disagree	Strongly Disagree	Uncertain	Missing Cases
In this hospital we believe in what we're doing.	38.98%	44.07%	1.69%	1.69%	11.87%	1.69%
Everyone in this hospital knows what it stands for.	11.86%	42.37%	15.25%	3.39%	27.12%	NA
This hospital provides me with an opportunity to excel professionally.	20.34%	44.07%	6.78%	1.69%	27.12%	NA
This hospital supports top quality work by investing in outstanding facilities and equipment	22.03%	49.15%	1.69%	22.03%	25.42%	1.69%
In this hospital, there is respect for the role and responsibilities of physicians.	32.20%	50.85%	3.39%	1.69%	10.17%	1.69%
There's a family feeling in this hospital.	15.25%	45.76%	11.86%	10.17%	16.95%	NA
This hospital allows me to do things that I find personally satisfying.	15.25%	62.71%	1.69%	5.08%	15.25%	NA
This hospital really cares about me as a person.	15.25%	47.46%	8.47%	5.08%	23.73%	NA
I'm encouraged to make suggestions about how the hospital can be more effective.	23.73%	52.54%	10.17%	6.78%	6.78%	NA
I take pride in being part of this hospital.	35.59%	50.85%	1.69%	1.69%	10.17%	NA
In this hospital we hear more about what physicians do right than the mistakes they make.	16.95%	57.63%	10.17%	3.39%	10.17%	1.69%
Communication within this hospital is very informal and frequent.	27.12%	52.54%	10.17%	3.39%	5.08%	1.69%
I've regretted that I chose to practice at this hospital.	6.78%	1.69%	28.81%	47.46%	16.56%	1.69%
This hospital stresses excellence and "doing it right."	16.95%	52.54%	5.08%	5.08%	20.34%	NA
This hospital makes me feel like I'm important.	11.86%	50.85%	15.25%	10.17%	11.86%	NA

database of similar physicians. The data in Table 8.1 shows a sample of questions that discern the perceptions of physicians, which demonstrate alignment in key factors that support physician partnerships.

Pie chart interpretation procedures (and any Likert scale interpretation) include analysis of variation. The degree of variation around each item determines whether the issue is good or bad in the eyes of the respondents. The easiest way to determine variation is to add the percentage of "agree" and "strongly agree." While there is no agreed upon absolute percentage of acceptability, if more than 70 percent (or more) of any group agrees or strongly agrees with a statement, then there is good alignment around that issue. Conversely, if the sum of the percentages in "uncertain," "disagree," and "strongly disagree" is equal to or greater than 50 percent, there is a significant problem. An "uncertain" score is considered negative. If leaders of change are not sure about something, the people below them in the organization cannot know. The whole purpose of completing organizational assessments is to determine the degree of alignment or misalignment around important intangible organizational issues.

Data on tangible issues. Collecting data on the tangible issues in healthcare most often focuses on the two, many times conflicting, issues of finance and quality. Administration typically emphasizes those aspects around "creating a bill and collecting payment; while keeping costs at a minimum." Physicians and other clinicians are more focused on meeting the patients' needs and working in a "hassle-free" work environment. Therefore, the tangible data can be subclassified into the business of healthcare and the mission or purpose of healthcare.

Each organization needs to isolate the data points, assessment instruments/methodology, and benchmarks. The principles for collecting tangible data are the same: validity and reliability of internal and external databases are essential. Multiple measures over time are necessary to show the degree of progress or regression. Most importantly, measurement must be viewed by those responsible for improvement as formative (that is, helpful) versus summative (judgmental).

CONCLUSION

We are what we measure. Remember, however, the wise thought from Peter Drucker: "Information is data with meaning." The role of leadership is to be sure that whatever is measured is relevant and meaningful to all those responsible for change and that all change management measurement protocols include data on both the tangibles and the intangibles. If you only measure the business aspects of healthcare, the mission will suffer. If you only measure the intangibles, the business may not survive.

For many years, it has been popular to say, "no margin, no mission." This mantra has been used to justify an extraordinary focus on the tangible, easy-to-measure economic aspects of healthcare delivery. Some executives, trustees, and consultants have used the no margin, no mission statement as a battle cry to radically reduce direct care staff and to put in place linear productivity models. The rationalization of margin before mission has damaged, and in some cases destroyed, the human spirit that underpins success in healthcare. We must become as skilled at measuring and managing the intangibles as we are at measuring the tangibles. And, we must *never* again use the statement "no margin, no mission." Replace this misguided mantra with, *"no balance, no business."* A board and executive mandate must be made to measure and manage the tangibles and the intangibles with the same discipline, precision and rigor. Without a clear strategy to measure and manage the intangibles, all business success will be short lived. It is in the spirit of those who deliver care that potential for long-term growth resides.

REFERENCES

Atchison, T. 1990. *"Turning Healthcare Leadership Around."* San Francisco: Jossey-Bass.

Braskamp, L. A., and M. M. Maehr. 1986. "The Healthcare Organizational Assessment Survey," A Spectrum Development Program. Champaign, IL: MetriTech.

Maher, M. M., and L. A. Branskamp. 1986. *The Motivation Factor: A Theory of Personal Investment.* Lexington, MA: Health.

Chapter Nine

A MODEL FOR
CHANGE MANAGEMENT

Good ideas are not adopted automatically. They must be
driven into practice with courageous patience.

Admiral Hyman Richover

T HE WAY CHANGE is managed with physicians and nonphysicians in healthcare settings varies widely in method
and results. Such wide variation along a success continuum has lead to skepticism and even cynicism. This book has attempted to present several ideas on ways to engage physicians and
nonphysicians in the process of performance improvement. Superficial and episodic interventions do not work and are counterproductive. Leaders must engage those affected by change in
order for a managed change process to work. The degree to which
the intangibles are measured and managed during the change
process will determine the success of any interventions.

Superficial and episodic attempts to change behavior need
to be replaced with deeper understanding and long-term, developmental processes. Leaders understand the importance of the

deeper dimensions that underlie success and that change is a process not an event. Humans are the most complicated factor in the change process, and no two workers will respond the same way to an intervention. Therefore, although a developmental model is useful in planning for change, in reality all organizational change is nonlinear. With these facts or caveats in mind, this chapter will describe a model that includes the critical intangibles that support any change attempts.

A MODEL FOR CHANGE

Quality healthcare is the prime objective of healthcare organizations. Quality, however, can be an allusive target. The developmental model for change begins with the notion that quality is an output. Figure 9.1(a) shows quality as both tangible and intangible. Figure 9.1(b) shows the importance of the bridge relationship between the tangibles and the intangibles. The space between these two domains is the "corporate soul." Another modification to the first grid is the belief that tangible quality is a function of intangible quality.

These grids reinforce that the essence of sustained improvement is intangible quality. The sequential and developmental process of intangible quality and the concomitant success in tangible quality can be shown in six triangles (see Figure 9.2).

These six triangles and 24 variables comprise the deeper dimensions of the managed change process. This process works for both expert and collective personalities with the caveat that experts (physicians) are more influenced by shared vision than shared values. These components are developmental in that each one depends on the existence of the previous one. The developmental sequence is as follows: leadership drives corporate culture; when there is a strong corporate culture, the personal investment can create a team spirit; and once there is a powerful sense of team, managing change will lead to intangible quality. Each of these developmental factors has four components.

Figure 9.1 Tangible and Intangibles

(a)

INPUTS

Tangible	Intangible
Cash	Mission
People	Values
Policy/Procedures	Vision
Strategy	Inspiration
Plant	Leadership Style
Information Systems	Recognition
Communications	Motivation

OUTPUTS

Tangible	Intangible
Profit	Culture
Market Share	Commitment
Products	Morale
Customer Satisfaction	Job Satisfaction
Growth	Team Spirit
Productivity	Pride/Joy/Trust
Quality	Quality

(b)

INPUTS

Tangibles	Corporate Soul	Intangibles
Cash	Meaning	Mission
People	Caring	Values
Policy/Procedures	Giving	Vision
Strategy		Inspiration
Plant		Leadership Style
Information Systems		Recognition
Communications		Motivation

OUTPUTS

Tangibles	Corporate Soul	Intangibles
Profit	Inner Peace of Purpose	Culture
Market Share		Commitment
Products		Morale
Customer Satisfaction	Joy	Job Satisfaction
Growth		Team Spirit
Productivity	Pride	Pride/Joy/Trust
Quality		Quality

"The soul is where the inner and outer world meets." —Novallis

"The Corporate Soul"* is the boundary between the Tangibles and Intangibles." —Atchison

*Adapted from: Awakening Corporate Soul, Klein and Izzo, 1998.

167

Figure 9.2   Sequential and Developmental Process of
Intangible Quality

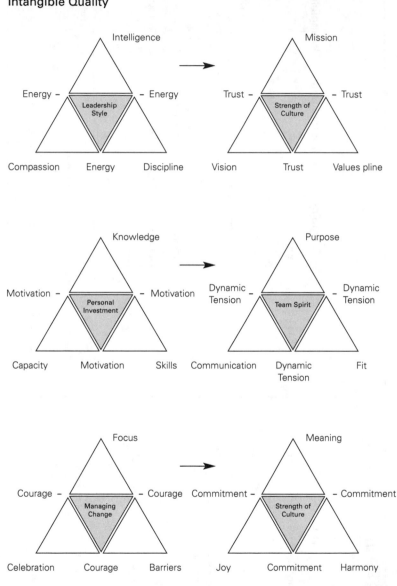

LEADERSHIP AND CORPORATE CULTURE

Leadership drives the corporate culture. All healthcare organizations are led in a way that produces the current reality. Everything about change management begins and ends with leadership. Chapter 6 discussed the dynamics of leadership and management and chapter 4 described the expert and collective cultures within the healthcare settings. Here, we discuss how strong corporate cultures underlie successful quality improvement programs and cost management processes because leadership has inspired followers who are committed, engaged, and enthusiastic. When quality is not improving and costs are not being managed because the workforce feels alienated, the problem is leadership. No amount of structural change will be effective. Figure 9.3 shows four characteristics of effective leaders: *intelligence, discipline, compassion, and energy.*

Leadership intelligence. The first leadership characteristic of intelligence is complicated. Individuals who possess several academic credentials are usually considered "intelligent." Gardner and Hatch (1989) posit that there are seven types of intelligence an individual may have to varying degrees: logical-mathematical, linguistic, musical, spatial, bodily-kinesthetic, interpersonal, and intrapersonal. Academic success requires logical-mathematical and linguistic skills. Leaders certainly need to be logical and possess good language skills. However, an argument could be made that these two skills alone make for good managers, not good leaders. To transcend from technical-managerial to inspirational leaders requires interpersonal and intrapersonal skills. High interpersonal and intrapersonal intelligence may be a greater component to effective leadership than logical-mathematical.

Jean Piaget, a researcher who studied intelligence, viewed intelligence in a biological framework. He believed that humans are intelligent to the degree they are able to adapt, adjust, and

Figure 9.3   Leadership Style

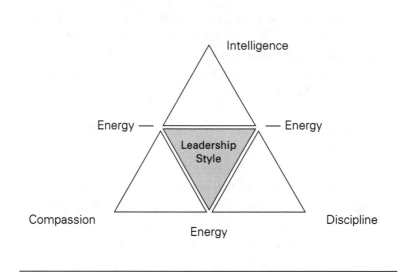

accommodate. Once again, we see intelligence as something greater than academic success or excellent recall skills. Intelligence in leaders is a combination of adaptability, realistic self-knowledge, and excellent interpersonal skills.

We hear these notions of intelligence reflected in the words of some preeminent organizational theorists. Tom Peters talks about "try it, fix it, do it" and "ready, fire, aim." Peter Senge asks us to change our "theories in use." Stephen Covey discusses the importance of "paradigm shifts." Leaders are challenged to maximize the adaptive intelligence and avoid an over dependence on the "things learned in school."

Leadership discipline. Leaders know that along with self-knowledge comes the belief that improvement is possible through concentrated effort and discipline. Impulsive behavior is avoided even in light of an unpredicted event. Leaders put episodes into a greater context to determine the best way to move forward. Their ability to discipline their minds and many times their bodies puts them in a position to cut through the noise and focus on the greater good for all.

Leadership compassion. Compassion is a unique element in the leader's repertoire. The notions of empathy, sensitivity, and genuine concern are very difficult to manifest in an industry that is constantly threatened. However, the most successful leaders are able to behave in ways that make followers feel like human beings not just "economic units." Compassionate leaders are not "wimps." Quite the contrary; leaders who possess adaptive intelligence, along with personal and professional discipline, are able to show genuine compassion. This occurs when all parties feel that they have been heard and the final decision was the best for everyone. Compassion allows leaders to do the right thing while protecting the self-worth of all involved.

Leadership energy. The final characteristic of effective leaders is energy. Leaders just do more. There is an important difference between being busy and the leadership trait of energy. Everyone in healthcare works very hard. However, much of the hard work is corrosive. Many of those who are the busiest are "burning out." Energy is the ability to work hard and become enriched in the process. Confucius once said: "Find a job that you love and you'll never work another day in you life." Leaders seem to thrive on the challenges that tire most others.

CORPORATE CULTURE

The special combination of intelligence, discipline, and energy are found in leaders who create strong corporate cultures. Without leadership, a single unifying corporate culture will not happen. Rather, the organization will default to multiple subcultures. To quickly review, corporate cultures have four elements: *mission,*

Figure 9.4   Strength of Culture

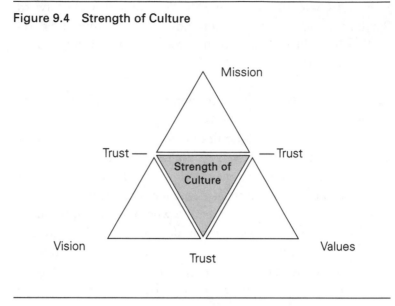

values, and vision, all held in place by *trust* (see Figure 9.4). Mission answers the question, Why do we exist? Values answer the question, What beliefs underlie our behavior? Vision answers the question, Where are we headed? Trust answers the question, Who is considered honest, open, and reliable? A strong corporate cultures exists to the extent the espoused values are displayed in everyone's behavior. Corporate cultures take a long time to create and are very resistant to change. However, when a strong culture is in place, the staff is free to personally invest in the organization. A weak culture is dominated by fear, uncertainty, and doubt.

PERSONAL INVESTMENT

Personal investment is an essential determinant in a successful change process. Maehr and Braskamp (1986) suggested that

Figure 9.5   Personal Investment

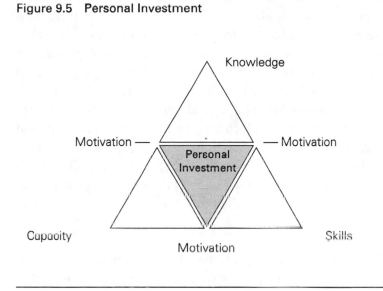

personal investment is the combination of "choice, persistence, continuing motivation, intensity and performance" (Maehr and Braskamp 1986, p. 10). The organizational staff must possess each of these variables in order to sustain change management processes. This critical intangible has four elements: *knowledge, skills, capacity, and motivation* (see Figure 9.5).

Knowledge and skills. Knowledge and skills must be in place at a high level for individuals to contribute to success. Fortunately, a great deal of time is spent on obtaining knowledge concerning a person's profession and the skills needed to execute the job requirements. Most continuing education programs target knowledge and skills development. One must assume competence in knowledge and skills for success to occur even at the minimum level. The challenge for leaders is in the other two elements, capacity and motivation.

Capacity. Capacity is a sensitive issue in these days of political correctness and "double speak." The truth is that all humans have limited potential, and to expect a person to exceed his or her capacity is counterproductive. Leaders must possess special skills to maximize everyone's capacity without creating expectations that are beyond an individual's ability. A myth in healthcare is that education and training are sufficient interventions to manage change. Actually, education is a necessary prerequisite but grossly insufficient condition to manage change. Knowing what is right does not ensure doing the right thing. The main factor is the capacity to execute. For example, understanding the physics behind dunking a basketball does not increase a person's vertical leap capacity.

Motivation. Motivation holds the other personal investment elements together. People must want to change before any intervention can be effective. The science of motivation is far too great for this book. However, the degree to which leaders understand why people behave the way they do will determine their success in change management. The basics of motivational theory are that all behavior is displayed for a purpose, and all behavior is learned. Because all behavior is learned, it can be unlearned or replaced with a different behavior. Behavior will change only when a new (replacement) behavior has more meaning or benefit to the individual. Chapter 8 discussed some of the motivational types that work in healthcare. The key is to match to motivational intervention to the person's needs.

Personal investment is a critical set of elements in this developmental model for change. No change can occur without individual effort. Unfortunately, many attempts at increasing personal investment fail because of the dependence on education as the strategy for change. The person's capacity to change and his or her level of motivation are the factors that determine success. Knowledge plus capacity plus motivation is the formula for increasing personal investment. Leaders need to spend at least

Figure 9.6   Team Spirit

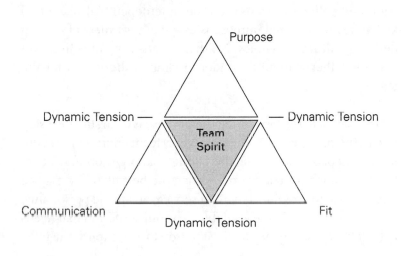

as much time and money on a group's capacity to change and its motivation to change as is spent on education. Personally invested staff are much more likely to engage in a team approach to change.

TEAM SPIRIT

Teamwork development is one of the major issues in today's literature addressing effective organizations. Teamwork is an outcome, not an input. You cannot "do team." Teamwork and team spirit are the results of four elements: *purpose, fit, communication, and dynamic tension* (see Figure 9.6).

Purpose. A common shared purpose is the first and most important element in creating a team. Our earlier discussion about the differences between expert and collective cultures (i.e., physicians and nonphysicians) made the point that teamwork is possible within each of these cultures. Separate metaphors were necessary to explain the different dynamics. Expert teams are like a golf team and collective teams are more interdependent like a basketball team. A shared purpose is essential regardless of the underlying cultural dynamics. Neither experts nor collectives will come together without an understanding of the reason for the team.

Fit the people to the task. Once the purpose is clear, the next step is to fit the right people to the task. Many team efforts fail because the wrong people are doing the wrong task. A person may be selected for a job for reasons other than the best fit. They may be selected because of title, length of service, an affable personality, or because they had time available. The only criterion that needs to be satisfied is: Are they the best person to accomplish the task?

Team communication. When the purpose is clear and the best people are fit to the task, the team will mature as a function of communication. During early development, new teams need to "hyper-communicate." The team needs to talk a great deal about purpose and role expectations. Open and honest communication will clarify misperceptions and avoid unnecessary conflict. Once a high level of teamwork exists, the communication style moves to "super-verbal." Great teams can anticipate their teammates' needs. For example, a new surgical team needs to talk about expectations. However, a surgical team that has been together a long time has developed an "anticipatory response." They know what their colleague needs without using words.

Teamwork and dynamic tension. Team communication reaches its highest level when dynamic tension exists. Dynamic tension is "loving combat." Great teams fight and argue about better ways to perform. The absence of personal attacks is also a characteristic of dynamic tension. Team members challenge each other

Figure 9.7   Managing Change

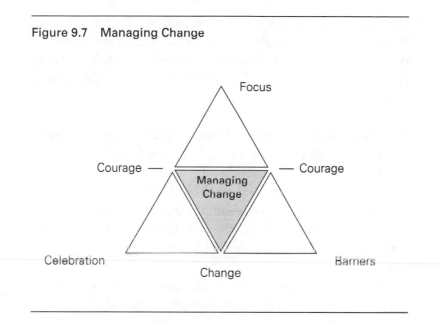

to perform at higher levels. The tension is dynamic because it improves the overall performance.

MANAGING CHANGE

High-performing teams make the change management process possible. The four elements of managing change are *focus, barrier analysis, celebration, and courage* (see Figure 9.7).

A clear team focus. Leaders have the ability to communicate their visions in ways that help others focus on specific changes. Clear focus drives all interventions. The focus for change must be something positive. Change cannot be managed when the target for change is to eliminate something undesirable. Telling someone to eliminate a behavior does not inform that person about the alternative behavior that would be acceptable. Negatives cannot be the focus for change. When the focus for change is a positive behavior, the negative behavior will disappear. Humans can only do one behavior at a time. Leaders always focus on the optimal performance.

Identifying barriers to success. Once the focus is clear, the barriers to success must be determined. These can be classified as personal, interpersonal, and structural.

Personal barriers to success are those that are embedded in the individual's personality. For example, one person might be very averse to risk taking, while another person might be unreasonably arrogant. Any idiosyncrasy that interferes with progress is a personal barrier.

Interpersonal barriers are those that emerge when two or more people interact. Typically these barriers are described as "communication problems." For example, if one group member intimidates another person, the change process will be contaminated. Structural barriers are any "man-made" problems. For example, human resources policies can be a barrier to change. The physical location of the organization is another common structural barrier.

Change management begins with clarification of the positive focus. The barriers to success are identified and classified. Some barriers can be eliminated and some can be reduced in terms of their potency. Some barriers, however, must be accepted. If one barrier to success is the way the government pays its bills, you just have to accept that and move on. If a human resources policy is a barrier, you may want to change the policy and eliminate the barrier. If location is a problem, you may wish to reduce the problem through video conferencing.

Celebration and recognizing progress. Celebration as an element of change management is often overlooked. Anytime a barrier to success is eliminated or reduced, a celebration must occur. Any recognition that highlights progress is a celebration such as a pat on the back, a thank you note, a pizza party, or a gift certificate. Lack of recognition is a significant error in the change management process. Interestingly, no change management process has failed because of too much recognition of success.

Courage to act. Focus, barrier analysis, and celebration are held together by courage. Warren Bennis' thoughts on courage were discussed earlier. Healthcare leaders today understand that the complexity of change issues demands courage to stay on the right course. Any systematic change process will offend at least one constituency. Courage in its simplest form is the capacity to act. Talking, analyzing, and processing are all good only if they lead to action.

INTANGIBLE QUALITY AND ORGANIZATIONAL PERFORMANCE

When all of the elements of leadership, corporate culture, personal investment, teamwork, and managing change are in place, the highest form of organizational performance can be reached. Intangible quality is rare in today's healthcare environment. The four elements of intangible quality are: *meaningful work, harmony, joy, and commitment* (see Figure 9.8).

Meaning and purpose. Throughout this book, we have emphasized the importance of meaning and purpose. The leader's role is to increase the performance of the staff for the benefit of quality care to the patients and excellent service to other customer groups. This is the noblest aspect of leadership. The best way to inspire the staff to increase performance is to create a work environment that provides meaning to the worker. Intangible quality starts with workers who work for more than a paycheck.

Figure 9.8   Intangible Quality

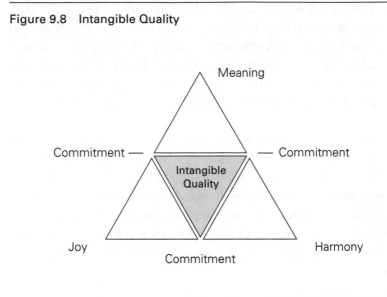

Harmony. When the work provides meaning and purpose to the staff, they witness harmony. The highest performing organizations complete multiple complex tasks effortlessly. Harmony does not mean "problem free." It means that is a "can do" attitude exists. It means blending. It means personal goals become secondary to a greater goal. A symphony orchestra is the classic analogy for harmony. Each instrument is played by an expert who understands how his or her performance creates the desired result. If each musician played what he or she wanted, when he or she wanted, the result would be chaos.

Joy. Joy is the third element of intangible quality. Chapter 10 speaks more to this important factor in organizational effectiveness. Joy comes from meaning and harmony. Joy and effort are not necessary related; simple tasks can be joyless and complex tasks can be joyful. It all goes back to meaning and the feeling of worth within the worker.

Commitment. The last element in this developmental model is commitment. Without commitment, you have nothing but an illusion. Commitment is the combination of pride, loyalty, and ownership. If you ask someone what parts of his or her life make them most proud, the answer usually will relate to a challenge that was met successfully. Humans want to take pride in their accomplishments and control the decisions that most affect them.

CONCLUSION

Change can be managed. The process described in this chapter incorporates the unique and unpredictable aspects of human behavior. Consequently, although the process is sequential and developmental, it is unpredictable. Some staff will respond quickly and positively. Others will be supportive but cautious. The skeptics will need considerable evidence that the change process is valid. There also exists in all organizations a small group of cynics who will never accept any change as good.

We have presented a sequence of 24 developmental elements that comprise a successful change management model. Each element needs to be factored into a process designed to launch or to sustain change. Change begins when leadership creates a strong culture. Change is then sustained when personally invested individuals become a team. The most important factor over time is when the managed change process has an underlying spirit of intangible quality. This model can be used as a roadmap or an audit tool. For as a planning tool the leader needs to develop strategies, tactics, and metrics for each element. For as an audit tool, if a change process is not working, find the element that is not in place and focus on it.

REFERENCES

Braskamp, L. A. and M. M. Maehr. 1986. "The Healthcare Organizational Assessment Survey," A Spectrum Development Program. Champaign, IL: MetriTech.

Gardner, H., and T. Hatch. 1989. "Multiple Intelligences Go to School: Educational Implications of the Theory of Multiple Intelligences." *Educational Researcher* 18.4–10.

Maher, M. M., and L. A. Branskamp. 1986. *The Motivation Factor: A Theory of Personal Investment.* Lexington, MA: Health.

Chapter Ten

RECOGNIZING THE ANSWERS

It is not because things are difficult that we do not dare; it is
because we do not dare that they are difficult.

Seneca

THE HEALTHCARE INDUSTRY is undergoing transformational change. Can the existing structures successfully
adapt, or will the inertia of entrenched power relationships render the current system progressively more disconnected
from the changing needs and expectations of society? First, organizations must be ready for change. Second, if the physician community cannot change and meet the expectations of society, they
risk losing professional status. We present some principles to follow in support of being the architect of your own future.

ORGANIZATIONAL VITAL SIGNS

Pascale et al. (1997) have written an article on leadership that
assesses what organizations must do if they are to successfully
transform themselves. They describe four attributes that define
potential for successful change:

183

- believing that you can make a difference;
- primarily identifying with the group;
- constructively managing conflict; and
- developing a learning organization.

BELIEVING YOU CAN MAKE A DIFFERENCE

Individual members of a group must feel that they can make a difference, effect change, and have a positive impact. If, on the other hand, they see circumstances as well beyond their capacity to have an influence, they will tend to be apathetic. The power of visionary leadership and the setting of "bold, audacious, hairy, goals" move individuals to create their own future (Collins and Porras 1997). This demands the emergence of strong leadership. James O'Toole (1995) writes that leadership is about ideas, about transcendent vision, and about the need to pursue a moral imperative. Successful leaders have passion for their vision and a passion to lead. They also have compassion for those they would presume to lead. To be effective, leaders highlight the best in their followers and give them hope. Their vision encompasses the needs and aspirations of their followers but will lead them to a place far better than they could have imagined on their own, actualizing the shared values of the workforce in pursuit of shared purpose that makes work matter. In these circumstances, people care about what they do and have fun doing it.

IDENTIFYING FIRST WITH THE GROUP

Each individual must hold his or her primary identity as a member of the group and not have primary allegiance to a segment of the group or a body outside the organization.

For example, physicians at the Mayo Clinic take pride first in being a member of the group and only secondarily to their professional or individual identity. They are selected for this cultural fit, expectations are clearly presented, and adherence to those expectations is demanded. They accept less salary for the privilege of belonging to a physician-directed, patient-focused organization that has a three-part mission: patient care, teaching, and research. Individual success is a derivative of collective success. Every other large physician organization that I am familiar with functions more like a condominium wherein each physician maintains a primary personal identity. They share space, referrals, and overhead, but collegiality overrides collaboration. The focus of each member is on personal needs and not on possibly subjugating those needs to an overriding collective vision.

OPENLY DEALING WITH CONFLICT

Change-ready organizations know how to deal with conflict. Avoidance is not the primary response to disagreement. Individuals are free to articulate their views and they do not duck the tough issues. The rapidly changing environment will continue to challenge organizations and require adaptations that will contribute to further changing the environment. It is a constant dialectic of change with individuals and organizations simultaneously effecting and being effected by the larger system within which they function. Diversity of opinion enriches discussion within the group and expands the realm of possible solutions. Conflict arising from difference of opinion in connection with a shared vision is something to strive for, not suppress. It may be used as a framework for contributing to a greater possibility for success.

DEVELOPING LEARNING ORGANIZATIONS

Change-ready organizations must be learning organizations. Remaining curious and vulnerable to new ideas is critical. Elements that characterize these successful organizations, influence organizational context and relationships, and cultivate an environment of creative change are:

- decentralization of decision making;
- diversification of people;
- dialog;
- sharing information;
- teamwork;
- aligned incentives;
- clarity of expectations;
- accountability;
- sharing rewards;
- intellectual capital;
- investing in the potential of the workforce; and
- unlayering organizational structure.

Successful organizations emphasize the intangibles of culture and employee pride (Pfeffer 1998). They coordinate many areas within the organization to reinforce a capacity for success. They simultaneously seek to focus individual, group, and organizational motivation and to invest in individual, interpersonal/interdepartmental, and organizational skills that serve to cohere the organization.

What do your organization's vital signs indicate?[1] Is it healthy, or is it in need of life-support? Are the constituents of your organization all in the same boat, rowing in unison to the cadence of shared vision and values, seeing their interdependency and how each contributes to the final direction and speed of the boat? Or do they row in response to their own dictates, creating turbulence, hindering performance, and maybe even going in circles?

THREATENED LOSS OF PHYSICIAN PROFESSIONAL STATUS

The overwhelming amount of change in healthcare over the past decade is beyond the control of any individual healthcare organization, physician, or physician group. The imposition of external demands has left the once proud and independent medical profession dependent on the whims of lawmakers, courts, popular opinions, fads, and ever-changing patient expectations. In truth, the failure of healthcare providers to heed the call to accountability invited many of the above intrusions of oversight and regulation.

Society has granted to physicians professional status.[2] O'Connor and Lanning (1992) define autonomy as the essence of professional status. Autonomy, the sine qua non of professionalism, is granted by society in exchange for meeting multiple expectations. These expectations, which are being challenged, include the following:

1. *Establishing criteria for admittance and licensure.* Standards of physician practice include credentialing and peer review. Because physicians have been reluctant to effectively perform these functions, external agencies have begun to establish criteria that define acceptable standards of practice.
2. *Holding members accountable for a level of performance higher than that required by legalities.* Physicians have failed to commit to outcome measurement and to identifying and applying processes of care that maximize outcomes. Indeed, our only experience with measurement is for judgment and not improvement.
3. *Committing to an ethical standard that holds service to others above economic self-interest.* The present climate of concern regarding fraud and abuse reflects society's growing suspicion that physicians may be making healthcare decisions more in deference to economics than patient welfare. Similarly, data showing wide variation in the application of healthcare resources have called into question the basis for clinical decision making.
4. *Defining how the profession should be organized and how services should be delivered.* Having decided that healthcare resources are no longer unlimited, society has asked for better value. Insurance companies, HMOs, legislatures, and the

business community are orchestrating the reorganization of health care delivery, in part because of physician unwillingness to positively respond to this need.

Because society believes that physicians fail to perform these functions, physicians risk losing autonomy and professional status. In some ways, the procedure-oriented physician who focuses on providing units of service independent from a holistic relationship with the patient is already acting as a tradesperson. Without concern for integration of the total outcome of care, they hold their relationship to a disease or a technology more important than the patient they are treating. Unless physicians respond to society's demands for collective accountability, externally imposed regulatory demands will replace autonomously held professional ethics as the basis for establishing criteria for adequate performance.

PRINCIPLES THAT CONTRIBUTE TO SUCCESS[3]

Some principles, guidelines, and approaches that enhance the likelihood that healthcare leadership can successfully navigate the whitewater of change include the following:

- act like an entrepreneur;
- focus primarily on people and not just finances;
- understand how to lead and manage change; and
- do not be afraid to reach out and be vulnerable.

ACT LIKE AN ENTREPRENEUR

Entrepreneurs are action-oriented persons who, when they recognize possible opportunities, act to pursue them (O'Connor and Bujak 2000). They take risks, act intuitively, and are not constrained by the current dominant paradigm. They do not say, "if only"; they imagine and experiment with "what if?" People are more likely to act themselves into new ways of thinking than to think themselves into new ways of acting (Pascale 1997). Unfortunately, in healthcare certain knowledge is often a precursor to action. Wayne Gretzky, a former star hockey player, is quoted as saying, "You miss 100% of the shots you don't take."

In the new economy, innovation and creativity are more important than perfectibility. It is more important to get it right, than not to get it wrong. Willingness is required to set the standards, and not just approximate someone else's. Pursuing a center of excellence concept, for example, seeks to benchmark the best of what is, leaving you vulnerable to what will be. In orthopedics, most organizations have initiated care paths and sought to enhance operational efficiencies, to reduce costs, and to preserve margins. In more innovative approaches, some have created joint camps that totally redesign the patient experience, delight the customer, and so enhance market share that they leave behind the approaches of yesterday. In the joint camp concept, patients move together along the path of preoperative preparation, surgery, recovery and rehabilitation, sharing a team concept, sharing expectations, and supporting and exhorting their fellow patients to achieve beyond the expected. A group identity is established and reinforced. Both the experience and the outcomes exceed those provided by traditional "centers of excellence."

FOCUS ON PEOPLE, NOT JUST FINANCES

Priorities need to shift to human resources (O'Connor and Bujak 2000). Organizational culture is one strategic advantage that cannot be copied. An investment in the competencies and knowledge of your workforce is the key to adaptability and success. Some are cautious about investing in the development of their employees, fearing that once trained they will leave for better opportunities. The only thing worse than investing in an employee who leaves is not investing in someone who stays. However, most organizations today continue to emphasize financial management capabilities and value costing and accounting skills over people skills. Far more critical to success is a willingness to nurture a culture of individual empowerment and accountability, cultivating relationships and managing context. Investing in human capital is critical.

Physicians must reassess their approach to patient care and integrate the efforts of all who are involved in creating patient outcomes. Healthcare has become far too complex and the amount of available information is too great to grasp. The interdependencies of variables are too complex for one person to know, and the enhanced outcomes that are consequent to ongoing measurement, process redesign, and interpersonal and interprofessional teamwork are too important to ignore through adherence to the outdated notion of the physician as the sole proprietor of patient care. Integrating and accessing necessary information, real-time measured feedback, and the expertise of all who can contribute to the best outcome possible are all necessary requirements to achieving the possible.

REACH OUT ... BE VULNERABLE

If the leadership and capital must come from the healthcare organization, healthcare executives must begin to understand physician culture and how to mobilize the physician community. We see little willingness on the part of healthcare executives to reach out to the physician community in a way that would lead to creative new partnerships. It is almost as if they are fearful of antagonizing this essential constituency. Usually, healthcare executives will hire one or more physician executives. The implicit expectation is that those physician executives "deliver their constituency," not only toward improved performance (translated: reduced cost of care), but also to a more friendly and less antagonistic posture toward the hospital. CEOs must recognize that physician executives are rejected by the majority of the medical staff and that the above stated goals are extremely difficult if not impossible to achieve. A direct approach on the part of the CEO to solicit the help and cooperation of the innovators and early adopters in his or her organization would be of more value. By exposing those individuals to new ideas and allowing them the space, resources, and time to test and modify those ideas, the CEO can fashion positive momentum for change, begin to build trust, and create the very objectives that he or she seeks. Very few physicians we know would refuse an expressed need for help. Saying to physicians, "I have a dream (necessarily one that encompasses the personal vision of the physicians in question) and this dream cannot be realized without your help and partnership," is a powerful way to begin the journey.

FINAL THOUGHTS

This book is fundamentally about the importance of intangibles as the factors that primarily determine the success and sustainability of organizations and relationships. We have stressed the critical role of vision, values, and measurement while emphasizing the interdependencies that exist within the provider community. For healthcare organizations to successfully partner with physicians they must coalesce into communities of shared meaning. Through joint pursuit of shared and transcendent purpose their interdependencies can come together in the expression of meaning and purpose in work and thereby restore and maintain a sense of joy and happiness in the workplace.

1. *It starts with vision.* Leadership is about authoring and communicating an inspirational and directional dream. Vision gives context and meaning to daily work. It highlights the best characteristics within the group, giving them hope and providing an image of a future state better than they could have imagined on their own. Creative tension is established when this idealized future is contrasted with an honest

assessment of current reality. Proactive choices designed to move the organization further toward achievement of the vision can then be made in the present. Decisions become understandable, and actions in the present take on context and meaning.

2. *Successful enterprises prioritize shared values.* Behaviors consistent with the group's shared values are identified, and those behaviors become the core competencies of the organization. In this way, work has meaning and purpose and becomes fun. The business strategy becomes a vehicle for the expression of the shared purpose and values of the organization. Purpose is the fundamental reason that the organization exists, and it remains immutable as long as that purpose is justified. It is the difference between the fundamental what and why of the organization as contrasted to the current how of the organization.

3. *Measurement is pivotal to success.* Without measurement there can be no management. Just deciding to measure something creates change in the direction intended, and not enough time is spent on deciding what should be measured. Do you measure what you value? Do you measure both the tangible and intangible aspects of the enterprise? For the enterprise to be successful, balance is essential.

4. *Success is in letting go.* Success lies not in establishing tighter controls, but in letting go. Successful leadership is about being a teacher and creating a learning organization. While the CEO may be in charge, he or she certainly is not in control. In a world where the future is unknowable, no one person, no administrative team can divine all the answers. However, the answers do lie within the collective wisdom of the organization. It is the job of leadership to influence context and relationships and to allow for the emergence of solutions that arise from within the collective workforce.

5. *Healthcare organizations and physicians are interdependent.*
   Although the nuts and bolts of managing organizations lie
   in an action orientation, an emphasis on people rather
   than finances, and the capacity to lead and manage change,
   success or failure will be determined in the ability to manage context and relationships. Healthcare organizations
   and their physicians are interdependent for their success.
   Creating successful partnerships at this level is the strategic
   imperative. Healthcare is a calling and not just a job.
   Reestablishing a sense of joy in the workplace requires
   the reaffirmation and rediscovery of meaning and purpose
   in work.

6. *The Four "l"s of life.* Stephen Covey and colleagues have
   written about the four "l"s of life: living, loving, learning,
   and legacy (Covey, Merrill, and Merrill 1994). The application to healthcare is clear: Living is about nurturing healing
   environments and creating and maintaining a sense of
   respect, pride, joy, and caring within the workplace. Loving
   is expressed in the commitment to interacting with others
   in transformational and not transactional ways. Attentive
   listening, clear communication, and refraining from acting
   on untested assumptions provide the foundation. Learning
   is about being alive in the present. It is about discovery,
   participation, and self-actualization. Legacy is about leaving
   this place better for our having been here. This is why the
   intangibles are so critical. If we could live life backwards,
   we would all acknowledge that what matters most is love
   and the quality of our relationships. Life is about being
   needed, being there for others, and pursuing a noble cause.
   It is never just about tangibles.

A lot is riding on our ability to successfully navigate the whitewater of change, the health of our patients, the health of our communities, and the very nature of our healthcare system—but the

most important—outcome is the soul and the spirit of those called to help heal others.

NOTES

1. These organizational vital signs are very consistent with the characteristics of a learning organization as outlined by Peter Senge in *The Fifth Discipline* (Senge 1990). They illustrate how the CEO may be "in charge," but is not "in control." For additional reading, see *Complexity and Management* by Ralph Stacey and colleagues. (Stacey, Griffin, and Shaw 2000). The authors seek to explain organizational reality, that is the realization that how things really get done in organizations in no way reflects formal organizational structure, process, or policy.

2. Refusing to respond to society's demands for measured accountability has invited the excessive regulatory overlay that is choking healthcare. The Institute of Medicine's report on adverse medical events, together with the documented variation with which medical care is practiced geographically, are stinging criticisms of healthcare's failure to commit to monitoring, measuring, and maximizing outcomes of care. The consequences are a progressive erosion of physician autonomy to the point where professional status is at risk.

3. Our principles for success emphasize action, people, and change management skills. As Peter Senge writes in *The Dance of Change*, "the new style of leadership is more inspiring than empowering, convincing than controlling, facilitating what might be rather than deciding what should be" (Senge 1999).

REFERENCES

Collins, J., and J. Porras. 1997. *Built to Last: Successful Habits of Visionary Companies.* New York: Harper Collins.

Covey, S., A. R. Merrill, and R. R. Merrill. 1994. *First Things First: To Live, to Love, to Learn, to Leave a Legacy.* New York: Simon and Schuster.

O'Connor, S. J., and J. A. Lanning. 1992. "The End of Autonomy? Reflections on the Postprofessional Physician." *Health Care Manage Review* 17(1): 63–72.

O'Toole, J. 1995. *Leading Change: Overcoming the Ideology of Comfort and the Tyranny of Custom.* San Francisco: Jossey-Bass.

Pascale R., M. Millemann, and L. Gioja. 1997. "Changing The Way We Change." *Harv. Bus. Review* (Nov-Dec) 76(6): 126–39.

Pfeffer, J. 1998. *The Human Equation: Building Profits by Putting People First.* Boston: Harvard Business School Press.

Senge, P. 1990. *The Fifth Discipline.* New York: Doubleday.

———. 1999. *The Dance of Change: The Challenges of Sustaining Momentum in Learning Organizations.* New York: Currency/Doubleday.

Stacey, R. D., D. Griffin, and P. Shaw. 2000. *Complexity and Management: Fad or Radical Challenge?* New York: Routledge.

About the Authors

Thomas A. Atchison, Ed.D., is president and founder of the Atchison Consulting Group, Inc., in Oak Park, Illinois. Since 1984, Dr. Atchison has consulted with healthcare organizations on managed change programs, team building, and leadership development. Dr. Atchison has written and been featured in a number of articles and audio and video tapes about motivation and managed change. He is the author of *Turning Healthcare Leadership Around* published in 1990. As an affiliate and faculty member of the American College of Healthcare Executives, Dr. Atchison has conducted seminars on partnering for change and recruiting and retaining effective employees. He earned his doctorate degree in Human Resource Development from Loyola University of Chicago.

Joseph S. Bujak, M.D., is vice president of medical affairs for the Kootenai Medial Center in Coeur d'Alene, Idaho, where he is responsible for performance improvement and outcomes measurement efforts. Dr. Bujak has extensive experience as a speaker, consultant, and facilitator working with physicians groups and healthcare organizations. Dr. Bujak is affiliated with the Kaiser Consulting Network and serves on the faculty of the American College of Healthcare Executives. He earned his medical degree from the University of Rochester in Rochester, New York.

ALSO FROM HEALTH ADMINISTRATION PRESS

**Medication Safety
and Cost Recovery
A Four-Step Approach
for Executives**
*Chip Caldwell, Jr. FACHE, and
Charles R. Denham, M.D.*

The core of this book is the 100-Day
Plan, a step-by-step model for reducing errors and recapturing costs.
Use the plan strategies to galvanize
your staff to reduce errors, establish
processes for attacking errors, evaluate how well interventions are working, and recover lost productivity.
The book also explores the many
factors that accelerate the reduction
of medication errors and those that
can slow improvement work. Get
your organization started by using
the tools for organizational assessment and planning contained in
the last chapter. These tools are also
available online in a workbook for-
mat that can be printed and copied
for use in your organization.

Order No. BKCO-1124, $56
Softbound, 200 pp, September 2001,
ISBN 1-56793-154-5
An ACHE Management Series Book

**Beyond Persuasion
The Healthcare Manager's Guide
to Strategic Communication**
Patricia J. Parsons

Communication is an important
management tool. It helps you build
and maintain the relationships—
with your patients, your staff, the
community, your board—that are
essential to your success. This book
will give you the knowledge and
attitude you need to communicate

effectively. Each chapter includes
many helpful checklists and examples that you can apply on the job.
Obtain practical tips and advice on
improving your interpersonal skills,
crafting effective memos and reports,
delivering presentations that engage
the audience, enhancing your rap-
port with your staff and board, and
confidently communicating with the
media.

Order No. BKCO-1122, $42
Softbound, 201 pp, June 2001
ISBN 1-56793-152-9

**Executive Excellence
Protocols for Healthcare Leaders,
Second Edition**
Carson F. Dye, FACHE

Technical skills do not ensure
leadership success. This book
describes the unwritten rules of
executive conduct that are critical
to your success as a healthcare
executive.

Issues covered include:

- Establishing relationships and
  strengthening credibility
- Making ethical choices
- Interacting with the executive
  team and board members
- Enhancing relationships with
  physicians
- Supporting increased diversity in
  the workplace
- Strengthening communications
  skills

Order No. BKCO-1111, $50
Softbound, 176 pp, 2000,
ISBN 1-56793-142-1
An ACHE Management Series Book

Prices do not include shipping and are subject to change.
To order, call (301) 362-6905 or purchase online at www.ache.org/hap.html